# Patient-Centered Care Series

## Series Editors

Moira Stewart,
Judith Belle Brown

and
Thomas R Freeman

# Eating Disorders

## A patient-centered approach

**Kathleen M Berg,**
**Dermot J Hurley,**
**James A McSherry**
**Nancy E Strange**
**and**
**'Rose'**

Radcliffe Medical Press

**Radcliffe Medical Press Ltd**
18 Marcham Road
Abingdon
Oxon OX14 1AA
United Kingdom

www.radcliffe-oxford.com
The Radcliffe Medical Press electronic catalogue and online ordering facility.
Direct sales to anywhere in the world.

---

British Library Cataloguing in Publication Data

A catalogue record for this book is available from the British Library.

ISBN 1 85775 922 2

Typeset by Aarontype Ltd, Easton, Bristol
Printed and bound by TJ International Ltd, Padstow, Cornwall

# Contents

# Series editors' introduction

The strength of medicine in curing many infectious diseases and some of the chronic diseases has also led to a key weakness. Some believe that medicine has abdicated its caring role and, in doing so, has not only alienated the public to some extent, but also failed to uphold its promise to 'do no harm'. One hears many stories of patients who have been technically cured but feel ill or who feel ill but for whom no satisfactory diagnosis is possible. In focusing so much attention on the nature of the disease, medicine has neglected the person who suffers the disease. Redressing this 20th century phenomenon required a new definition of medicine's role for the 21st century. A new clinical method, which has been developed during the 1980s and 1990s, has attempted to correct the flaw, to regain the balance between curing and caring. It is called a Patient-Centered Clinical Method and has been described and illustrated in *Patient-Centered Medicine: transforming the clinical method* (Stewart et al., 1995) of which the 2nd edition is being prepared for publication in early 2003. In the 1995 book, conceptual, educational and research issues were elucidated in detail. The patient-centered conceptual framework from that book is used as the structure for each book in the series introduced here; it consists of six interactive components to be considered in every patient–practitioner interaction.

The first component is to assess the two modes of ill health; disease and illness. In addition to assessing the disease process, the clinician explores the patient's illness experience. Specifically, the practitioner considers how the patient feels about being ill, what the patient's ideas are about the illness, what impact the illness is having on the patient's functioning and what he or she expects from the clinician.

The second component is an integration of the concepts of disease and illness with an understanding of the whole person. This includes an awareness of the patient's position in the lifecycle and the social context in which they live.

The third component of the method is the mutual task of finding common ground between the patient and the practitioner. This consists of three key areas: mutually defining the problem, mutually defining the goals of management/treatment, and mutually exploring the roles to be assumed by the patient and the practitioner.

The fourth component is to use each visit as an opportunity for prevention and health promotion. The fifth component takes into consideration that each encounter with the patient should be used to develop the helping relationship;

the trust and respect that evolves in the relationship will have an impact on other components of the method. The sixth component requires that, throughout the process, the practitioner is realistic in terms of time, availability of resources and the amount of emotional and physical energy needed.

However, there is a gap between the description of the clinical method and its application in practice. The series of books presented here attempts to bridge that gap. Written by international leaders in their field, the series represents clinical explications of the patient-centered clinical method. Each volume deals with a common and challenging problem faced by practitioners. In each book, current thinking is organized in a similar way, reinforcing and illustrating the patient-centered clinical method. The common format begins with a description of the burden of illness, followed by chapters on the illness experience, the disease, the whole person, the patient–practitioner relationship and finding common ground, including current therapeutics.

The book series is international, to date representing Norway, Sweden, Canada, Australia, New Zealand and the USA. This is a testament to the universality of the values and concepts inherent in the patient-centered clinical method. The work of not only the authors, but others who have studied patients, has reinforced a virtually identical series of six components (Little *et al.*, 2001; Stewart, 2001). We feel that there is an emerging international definition of patient-centered practice which is represented in this book series.

The vigor of any clinical method is proven in the extent to which it is applicable in the clinical setting. It is anticipated that this series will inform further development of the clinical method and move thinking forward in this important aspect of medicine.

Moira Stewart PhD
Judith Belle Brown PhD
Thomas R Freeman MD, CCFP

# References

Little P, Everitt H, Williamson I *et al.* (2001) Preferences of patients for patient-centred approach to consultation in primary care: observational study. *BMJ.* **322**(7284): 468–72.

Stewart M (2001) Towards a global definition of patient-centred care. *BMJ.* **322**(7284): 444–5.

Stewart M, Brown JB, Weston WW *et al.* (1995) *Patient-Centered Medicine: transforming the clinical method.* Sage Publications, Thousand Oaks, CA.

# Foreword

It would be difficult to find a better example of the importance of the patient-centered approach than eating disorders. The essence of the patient-centered clinical method is the attempt by the clinician to enter the patient's world, to see the illness through the patient's eyes and to reconcile this perspective with the clinician's analysis of the illness. The importance of reaching this common ground has been demonstrated in many studies showing improved outcomes of illness. The patient-centered approach is desirable in all disorders. In eating disorders, it is not only desirable but essential. Unless some common ground can be attained, the clinician's efforts are unlikely to be effective, but in few disorders is achieving common ground more difficult. The cognitive distortions that are such a feature of eating disorders make it unlikely that any common ground will be attainable until the clinician has earned the trust of the patient, and this may take a long time, given the suspicion of therapists that is so often a feature of these disorders.

In few conditions is teamwork more essential. Common ground is important, not only between clinician and patient, but also between team members. It is not enough for the patient to be serially referred from one to the other. The clinicians are not a team unless they talk to each other and respect each other's knowledge and perspective. This book is written by members of a team who have collaborated for many years in the care of patients with eating disorders. They all speak from extensive experience and have many wise things to say. The book is also enriched by accounts written by patients themselves: personal memoirs, case reports, and qualitative studies. One whole chapter, a very moving one, is a patient's story told by herself: Rose's story. There can be no better way of developing the necessary empathy than reading these stories. Giving other patients' stories is important also, since eating disorders are heterogeneous and patients differ in their ideas, emotions, expectations and experience.

The authors represent the four disciplines most involved with these patients: family medicine, clinical psychology, dietetics and social work/family therapy. The family physician or pediatrician is often the person to make the diagnosis and to bring together the team. He or she has probably known the patient prior to her illness, and may well have cared for her family. He or she will be the team member most concerned with the bodily consequences of the disorder. The psychologist addresses the complex psychological factors, which can contribute to the onset of the disorder and also to its persistence; factors such as low self-esteem, disturbance of body image, cognitive distortions, distrust of professionals and resistance to therapy. The dietitian works with the patient in setting goals for the normalization of eating habits, meeting of nutritional needs, and attainment of optimal weight. Once the goals are set by mutual agreement, the dietitian helps the patient to achieve them; often a long and difficult process involving changes in harmful eating patterns and attitudes to food. The social worker/family therapist is especially concerned with family relationships. An eating disorder places enormous stresses on family members. Often they have great difficulty dealing with behavior they do not understand and which they see as irrational. Struggles may arise over such issues as meal times and the disappearance of food. When their attempts to control the problem are unsuccessful they become desperate for help and support. The social worker/family therapist can meet these needs and help the family to play a significant role in the patient's recovery.

Besides exploring the patient's experience, understanding the whole person, enhancing the clinician–patient relationship and trying to reach common ground, the patient-centered method enjoins the clinician to 'be realistic'. Usually, this is interpreted as making appropriate use of limited resources, such as the time available for a consultation. Eating disorders give a different meaning to the word 'realistic'. Here, the reality is the long duration of the illness and the patience and perseverance required in the clinician. This is realism that is pleased with small steps and tolerant of backward ones.

This book is a rich source of wisdom and insight.

IR McWhinney
*July 2002*

# About the authors

**Kathleen M Berg** PhD, CPsych is a psychologist in private practice in London, Ontario. Dr Berg has been engaged in both individual and group treatment of eating disorders since 1983. She is on the Board of Directors of the Eating Disorders Association of London and is an adjunct faculty member of the Department of Psychiatry at the University of Western Ontario. She has, in the past, been on staff at the Student Development Centre at UWO, taught courses for the Department of Psychology and served as psychological consultant for Huron College. Dr Berg's research interests have included the prevalence of eating disorders, the heterogeneity of behavioral and cognitive symptomatology in bulimia nervosa, and the development of a community handbook on detection, treatment and coping strategies for eating disorders. She has conducted numerous professional and educational workshops on eating disorders and body image, and has been a long-time advocate of a client-centered approach to treatment, education and prevention.

**Dermot J Hurley** MSW, RSW is a clinical social worker with 20 years' practice experience with children and adolescents. He is Director of the Family Therapy Program, Division of Child and Adolescent Psychiatry, London Health Sciences Centre. He lectures in social work at King's College, London and is Assistant Professor of Psychiatry (Part Time), University of Western Ontario. Dermot has been involved in the development of innovative programs in the London area for many years for children of separation and divorce, and has a special interest in the therapy of grieving and traumatized children. His areas of specialty include child and adolescent psychotherapy, marital and family therapy and systemic therapy for families with an eating disorder.

**James A McSherry** MB, ChB is a 1965 medical graduate of the University of Glasgow. He is a family physician in London, Ontario and a Professor in the Departments of Family Medicine and Psychiatry at the University of Western Ontario, and Chief of Family Medicine at London Health Sciences Centre. He founded the Canadian Primary Care Eating Disorders Association in 1998 and is editor of its newsletter. He has been President of the Eating Disorders Association of London since 1993. His interest in eating disorders originated from his work as Director of the Student Health Service at Queen's University, Kingston, Ontario between 1981 and 1993.

**Nancy E Strange** BA, RD is a registered dietitian at the Children's Hospital of Western Ontario, part of the London Health Sciences Centre. She obtained a BA with a major in foods and nutrition from the University of Western Ontario and completed a dietetic internship at Brantford General Hospital. She is a member of The Dietitians of Canada and The College of Dietitians of Ontario. With over 25 years' experience as a member of multidisciplinary teams working with both adolescents and adults with eating disorders, she works in both inpatient and outpatient settings and enjoys the challenges these patients and their families provide. She has made frequent presentations on eating disorders and their treatment to audiences of health professionals, parents and high school students.

# Acknowledgments

The authors are deeply indebted to Renata Tichy for valuable consultations provided during all phases of the writing of this book.

Additionally, they offer their gratitude to Jean Hood for her skill, patience and perseverance in the preparation of the manuscript.

This book is dedicated to the memory of

**Dr James McSherry**

whose vision, wisdom and commitment to a patient-centered
understanding and treatment of eating disorders led to the writing
of this book,

and to the memory of

**Jean Hood**

whose tireless efforts and dedication were a constant source of
support to the authors.

# Introduction

*James A McSherry*

What is an 'eating disorder' and why do we need a 'patient-centered' approach to management?

To the person in the street, the term 'eating disorder' probably means anorexia nervosa or bulimia nervosa, unusual conditions where affected persons display odd behaviors such as food refusal, binge eating and self-induced vomiting in a poorly understood drive for thinness.

To the person affected by an eating disorder, the condition involves a set of values, beliefs and behaviors that have deep personal meaning, relevance and significance for the affected individual. That person's eating disorder can only be understood within the context of his or her unique individual experience.

Health professionals tend to view eating disorders from a perspective that reflects their orientation in specific disciplines, e.g. medicine, psychiatry, psychology, social work and nutrition. Their approach to the person with an eating disorder is, therefore, often limited by the relatively narrow vantage point of a particular professional ethos and culture, when understanding the whole patient requires a more broadly based multidimensional perspective on what the condition means to the affected individual and his or her significant relationships.

Without that multidimensional approach, the numerous and complex factors that are fundamental to the initiation and maintenance of an eating disorder may go unrecognized and unchallenged. If an eating disorder is no more than a mood disturbance to the psychiatrist, malnutrition to the dietitian, a cognitive distortion to the psychologist, a dysfunctional family to the social worker or family therapist, an electrolyte imbalance to the family physician or internist, then the condition becomes misrepresented as its shadow rather than its substance. The larger epiphenomenology is seen as more important than the central issue.

The term 'multidimensional' is deliberately used here in preference to 'multidisciplinary'. Healing for the person with an eating disorder often requires the services of professionals from a variety of health disciplines, but those services may be more problematic than healing unless healthcare providers operate from a shared basic philosophy. Seeing the whole person behind the diagnostic label, appreciating the illness experience and developing an integrated understanding of the dimensions of an illness and what it means to the individual patient all require an approach that goes well beyond the conventional biomedical model that has dominated medical thinking for so many years.

This book seeks to offer insights into the values and beliefs that mould attitudes and behaviors into the conditions of physical, physiological and psychological dysfunction that we recognize as eating disorders. It does so in a way that is based on the principles of patient-centered medicine, principles that become operational as a shared philosophy of care in which the contributions of each member of a multidisciplinary care team are harmonized in the best interests of each patient.

All six components of the patient-centered method have special relevance to the care of patients with eating disorders, as the following work, comprising the collaborative efforts of five individuals, will show. Four of them, a family physician, a clinical psychologist, a registered dietitian and a social worker, are clinicians actively involved in helping persons and families who battle with eating disorders. They have considerable experience of working in teams, in both formal, institution-based and informal community-based settings and are committed to a patient-centered approach to patients with eating disorders. The fifth is a person in recovery from an eating disorder who has generously and courageously contributed her own story to illuminate the illness experience.

Because over 90% of those with eating disorders are female, the feminine pronoun is used throughout the book. However, the authors respectfully acknowledge the experiences of a growing number of males who suffer from eating disorders.

The case studies described in this book have been thoroughly disguised to preserve confidentiality.

# Magnitude of the problem

*James A McSherry*

Eating disorders are frequently assumed to be a modern disease whose origins lie in an overstressed, prosperous world. A world where societal pressures to be slim have created epidemic preoccupation with size and shape among young women. Standards of female beauty do change from time to time, perhaps in response to changing social conditions and food availability. The glamorized 'ideal' female shape, as defined by Western cultural standards, has changed visibly and measurably in modern times. A 1980 study found that *Playboy* centrefolds and Miss America contestants had become progressively lighter in weight and more 'tubular' in appearance over a period of 20 years, setting standards that are genetically and biologically impossible for the vast majority of women (Garner *et al.*, 1978). In a curious paradox, the average woman's weight has been increasing at a rate almost exactly matched by the decline in the weights of our cultural icons. There is an inverse relationship between female body weight and socioeconomic status in contemporary Western society; the higher a woman's socioeconomic status the more likely she is to be thin and to project an image of success, self-assurance and strength. We live in a culture of 'weightism', where to be overweight is to be devalued as somehow lacking in moral fibre and disadvantaged in social and employment-related settings.

It hasn't always been so. To be overweight when others are starving indicates a certain place on the social ladder of power and prestige, it has been argued, while being slim in an age of plenty indicates a superior degree of fastidiousness and an aloofness from the common herd. Many celebrated beauties of former ages, if alive today, would find themselves encouraged to attend an obesity clinic or 'fat farm' since their tendency to what we would regard as overweight runs contrary to modern taste. There is a certain face validity to this viewpoint, but the truth is that food refusal has been documented as a female assertiveness response for many centuries in times of plenty and in times of want. It is our interpretation of this behavior and our definition of the core attributes of a disordered belief system that has changed the way we look at such a phenomenon.

An understanding of that disordered belief system and the role it plays in the lives of people affected by an eating disorder is fundamental to any attempt to help those people overcome conditions that have serious consequences for their physical and psychological well-being.

The *Diagnostic and Statistical Manual* (American Psychiatric Association, 2000b) is the standard reference book that classifies psychiatric conditions and defines the criteria by which they are diagnosed. Usually referred to as DSM, it is now in its fourth edition. DSM-IV-TR describes three specific eating disorders: anorexia nervosa, bulimia nervosa and 'eating disorder not otherwise specified'. Anorexia nervosa and bulimia nervosa are the best known of the eating disorders because, as diagnostic categories, they define serious abnormalities of eating attitudes and behaviors that have important consequences for the physical and mental health of affected individuals. However, they fail to capture the extent to which less severe forms of both conditions appear in any given population and 'eating disorder not otherwise specified' (EDNOS) is the term used to describe the situation where an individual presents with features highly suggestive of an eating disorder, but lacking the severity or chronicity to justify a diagnosis of anorexia nervosa or bulimia nervosa.

# Diagnostic criteria

The basic DSM-IV-TR (American Psychiatric Association, 2000b) diagnostic criteria for anorexia are:

- refusal to maintain a normal body weight for age and height, or failure to make expected weight gains at times of growth and physical development
- fear of gaining weight or becoming fat
- an abnormal body image
- cessation of menstrual periods in women who are not using any external source of estrogen, e.g. oral contraceptives.

Persons affected by anorexia nervosa believe themselves to be fat and overweight despite all objective evidence to the contrary. Bulimic and restricting subtypes of anorexia nervosa are recognized. Patients with the restricting subtype drastically reduce their daily calorie intake without binge eating, purging or using laxatives or diuretics on anything other than an occasional basis. Their eating attitudes and behaviors often have an overt obsessive–compulsive flavor with elaborate rituals around preparation of food that is frequently offered to others, but never consumed by the affected individuals. Patients with the bulimia nervosa subtype have frequent eating binge/purge episodes. Some patients with anorexia nervosa purge without binge eating, at least by objective measures.

Bulimia nervosa is characterized by:

- recurrent episodes of uncontrollable binge eating followed by such inappropriate attempts at compensation as self-induced vomiting, misuse of laxatives and excessive exercise
- preoccupation with size, shape and weight.

Eating binges are episodes of rapid consumption of large quantities of food over relatively short periods of time and should occur at least twice a week for at least three months to satisfy the DSM-IV criteria. Once triggered, eating binges are perceived as beyond the affected individual's personal control until they are terminated by running out of food, experiencing intolerable physical discomfort, involuntarily vomiting or some kind of social interaction that produces an enforced distraction. There is evidence for a significant overlap of abnormal attitudes and behaviors between anorexia nervosa and bulimia nervosa (Bulik *et al.*, 1997) since as many as 50% of patients with anorexia nervosa may develop bulimic symptoms and patients with bulimia nervosa may display anorexic symptoms.

# Atypical eating disorders

The DSM-IV category 'EDNOS' is essentially a classification that captures individuals whose behaviors are clearly abnormal and clinically significant, but fail to match exact diagnostic criteria for anorexia nervosa and bulimia nervosa, the so-called 'atypical eating disorders'. Diagnostic criteria are artificial concepts at best, arbitrary constructs that define conditions of unequivocal severity where abnormal eating attitudes and behaviors are clearly pathological and have recognizable consequences that are harmful to the affected person. The 10th edition of the World Health Organization's International Classification of Diseases (ICD-10) identifies 'atypical eating disorders' as those conditions in which the general features support a diagnosis of anorexia nervosa or bulimia nervosa, but one or more of the key features are missing or present only in minor degree.

# Frequency and outcome

The lifetime prevalence of anorexia nervosa in women is between 0.5% and 3.7% (Garfinkel *et al.*, 1995; Walters and Kendler, 1995) and between 1.1% and 4.2% for bulimia nervosa (Garfinkel *et al.*, 1995; Kendler *et al.*, 1991).

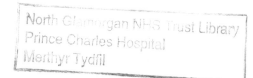

Anorexia nervosa appears to be uncommon outside Western society, but immigrants from less-developed to more-developed countries are more likely to develop eating disorders than their sisters who stayed in their countries of origin (Vandereycken and Hoek, 1992). The observation that the onset of an eating disorder frequently coincides with puberty suggests that young women may misinterpret their changing shape as 'getting' fat and engage in dieting behavior in an attempt to regain their former 'slim' androgenous shape. It is also possible that young women may find themselves uncomfortable in their new role as developing adults and feel threatened by a sexuality with which they have not previously had to deal. Weight loss and regression of secondary sexual characteristics effectively resolve these issues. Both anorexia nervosa and bulimia nervosa occur most often in college and university women, but are far from exclusive to them (Marciano *et al.*, 1988). Primary care physicians recognize only 40% of patients with anorexia nervosa, and bulimia nervosa in only 11% (Hoek, 1991). The category EDNOS recognizes that many women suffer from disorders of eating attitudes and behaviors that cannot be assigned to a specific diagnostic category, but are, nevertheless, important causes of psychological distress, physical health problems and reduced quality of life for those affected.

The following 'prayer' was given to the author (McSherry, 1984) by one of his patients and seems to express many of the frustrations experienced by such women.

# The Prayer of the Pleasing Child

I feel fat.
Yesterday I felt fat,
but today I ate.
Why does my stomach rule my mind?
I just want to stop eating, period.
No food,
Just quit . . . cold turkey.
That is a bad expression for a dieter.
Tomorrow I have to force my body into submission.
I have to love myself.
I hate myself when I eat,
So, if I don't eat,
Even though it hurts,
I love myself.
Oh, I feel so gross!
If only I could peel myself like a banana,

Release the true me,
Under the layer of flab
which stops me from interacting, from loving, from living.
I have to stop eating.
Chains we cannot see,
Come release us, Lord,
From chains we cannot see,
But how we feel them!
I want to be a pleasing child.
Until that final day,
God please help me get control again.

The common theme in eating disorders is preoccupation with body weight and shape, often accompanied by dietary faddism with unusual food preferences. Depressed mood is associated with eating disorders in 50% to 75% of affected individuals (Braun *et al.*, 1994; Hamli *et al.*, 1991; Herzog *et al.*, 1992). Women are affected between six to nine times more frequently than men, except in adolescence, where 19%–30% of eating disorders patients are male (Fosson *et al.*, 1987; Hawley, 1985; Higgs *et al.*, 1989).

A review of 68 outcomes studies published between 1953 and 1986 (Steinhausen, 1995) analyzed data from 3104 patients who had been followed for periods between one and 33 years. Forty-nine percent of patients affected by anorexia nervosa returned to normal eating behavior, while 60% returned to normal weight and menstruation. Over 40% of anorexia nervosa-affected persons could be said to have recovered, over 30% were improved and 20% had a persistent chronic illness. The overall mortality was 5%, although the studies individually reported mortality rates of 0% to 21%. Positive outcomes were found to be dependent on such variables as personality, a conflict-free relationship with parents, early treatment, risk avoidance, emotional restraint and conformity to authority. Conversely, vomiting, bulimia nervosa, profound weight loss, chronicity, impulsiveness, lack of self-esteem and distrust of others were indicators of a generally poor prognosis.

About 50% of those struggling with bulimia nervosa recover with cognitive behavioral therapy, about 30% have a persistent, less severe but chronic illness and 20% have a persistent condition that is resistant to therapy (Hsu, 1995). Although 30% of persons with normal weight bulimia nervosa have a previous history of anorexia nervosa, relapse is infrequent (Hsu, 1995).

# Risk factors

Do individuals with already abnormal eating attitudes and behaviors or disturbed body image actually select particular vocations and pursuits that seem to be associated with a high prevalence of eating disorders? Is it the occupation or the hobby that produces the disorder? The answers are not entirely clear. Known factors that place individuals at increased risk for developing an eating disorder include dieting behavior, use of hazardous weight-loss measures, childhood obesity (Cooper, 1995b), sexual abuse (Welch and Fairburn, 1994), medical conditions that focus attention on nutrition and weight control, e.g. diabetes mellitus (Peveler, 1995), androgen excess syndromes, etc. (McSherry, 1990). Additionally, membership in predisposed vocational groups such as models, ballet dancers, skaters, gymnasts, wrestlers, jockeys, flight attendants, athletes, etc. increases risk (Mickalide, 1990).

Abnormal eating attitudes and behaviors, pathological weight-control measures, even eating disorders themselves are common in female athletes (Sundgot-Borgen, 1993), with the caveat that the presence of a clinically significant eating disorder will prejudice the likelihood of an affected person reaching the highest levels of performance.

# The meaning of words

The term 'anorexia nervosa', Latin for 'nervous loss of appetite', was introduced into general use by Sir William Withey Gull, an English physician, in 1873. It is one of modern medicine's greatest misnomers since patients struggling with anorexia have not lost their appetites, they are actually engaged in its rigorous suppression. Failure to understand this basic concept is a major obstacle to any understanding of the individuals affected by the disorder. The word 'bulimia' was introduced into the English language by Dr Samuel Johnson in his famous Dictionary. It means 'ox-eating' and was used by Xenophon (c. 428–354 BC) in his *Anabasis* to describe the voracious eating behaviors of his soldiers after a long period of semi-starvation (Parry-Jones and Parry-Jones, 1995).

# The history of eating disorders

Eating disorders are modern clinical concepts based on diagnostic criteria of relatively recent origin. It is, therefore, difficult to make retrospective diagnoses except in unusually well-documented cases since the kind of medical assessment that would exclude other conditions is not available. However, it is highly likely that eating disorders, or at least instances of prolonged food refusal with binge eating and self-induced vomiting, were well established, if poorly understood, features of the health landscape long before Sir William Gull coined the term 'anorexia nervosa' in 1873 (Gull, 1874). Society has from time to time interpreted food refusal in a variety of ways and developed responses that have been appropriate to contemporary knowledge about health and the human psyche. Indeed, the 19th century appears to have marked a cultural divide when fasting became a medical problem rather than, as anorexia mirabilis, an object of awe and an important sign of piety. Additionally, 'hunger strikes' are a time-honored means of social protest or civil disobedience.

St Wilgefortis (Lacey, 1982) was the Christian daughter of a 9th century pagan king of Portugal. Betrothed to a Saracen king of Sicily, she began to fast in order to make herself as unattractive as possible to a future spouse, as she had already decided to take Holy Orders and enter a convent. She succeeded to the point that her suitor refused to marry her when at last they met. Her father, it is said, was so furious that he had her crucified. She still exists in European legend and has become the patron saint of women who wish to rid themselves of an unwanted spouse. Known variously as St Uncumber, St Liberata or St Livrade, she is usually portrayed nailed to a cross or as a young woman with a beard, hence her fame as the 'bearded female saint'. The beard is likely an artistic interpretation of the lanugo that commonly occurs in women who are emaciated for any reason. She clearly did not have anorexia nervosa as we understand it today, as her fasting was deliberately undertaken in full knowledge of its harmful effects.

Robert Willan, a London physician and dermatologist, described *A Remarkable Case of Abstinence* in 1790 (Hunter and MacAlpine, 1963) and is usually accorded priority in describing anorexia nervosa in males. A young man 'of studious and melancholic mind' undertook 'a severe course of abstinence' because of 'pains in the stomach and a constant sensation of heat internally' and 'some mistaken notions in religion'. The studious young man consumed only sips of water and kept himself busy copying and annotating a bible. He was 'emaciated to a most astonishing degree ... a most ghastly appearance' and Willan described him as looking like a skeleton that had been prepared by drying all the muscles. He exhibited 'an enthusiastic turn of mind, nearly bordering on insanity'. Dr Willan's studious and melancholic young man died of exhaustion after 60 days.

John Reynolds published *A Discourse Upon Prodigious Abstinence Occasioned By the Twelve Months Fasting of Martha Taylor, the Famed Derbyshire Damosell* in 1669 (Hunter and MacAlpine, 1963) but Dr Richard Morton (Morton, 1694) was the first to note the syndrome of loss of appetite, amenorrhea and extreme wasting without any recognizable evidence of known disease. Dr Morton's *Phthisiologia; or a treatise of consumptions*, a 1694 translation of his 1689 work *Phthisiologia, seu exercitationes de phthisi tribus libris comprehensae. Totumque opus variis historiis illustratum*, described 'Nervous Atrophy, or Consumption' in a young woman, 'Mr Duke's Daughter in St Mary Axe' who in 1684:

and the Eighteenth year of her Age, in the Month of July fell into a total suppression of her Monthly Courses from a multitude of Cares and Passions of her Mind, but without any of the symptoms of the Green-Sickness following upon it. . . . her Appetite began to abate, and her Digestion to be bad; her Flesh also began to be flaccid and loose, and her looks pale, with other Symptoms usual in an Universal Consumption of the Habit of the Body.

Mr Duke's daughter consulted Dr Morton after she had been ill for two years and only then because she was having 'frequent Fainting Fits'. Morton described her appearance as 'like a Skeleton only clad with skin', and found it remarkable that she exhibited no symptoms or signs that would suggest a recognizable medical condition. Mr Duke's daughter died three months later.

Dr Morton was more successful in the case of 'The Son of the Reverend Minister Steele', a young man who began to fast when he was 16 years of age, 'pining away more and more, for the space of two Years'. Told to give up his studies, go to the country, take up riding and drink plenty of milk, he 'recovered his Health in great measure', giving Dr Morton not only priority in describing anorexia nervosa in a male, but also in recording the earliest successful treatment.

Mary Stewart, perhaps better known as Mary Queen of Scots, was born in 1542 and died by beheading in 1587. Her father died a few days after she was born and her mother sent her to France from Scotland for safety when she was five years of age. Mary was raised at the court of Henry II and her medical history is known in surprising detail thanks to the efforts of the various ambassadors who provided their own sovereigns with regular intelligence from France. It is known she had measles when she was five years of age, rubella when she was seven, a dental abscess when she was 12, both dysentery and malaria when she was 14, and smallpox when she was 15.

Additionally, she had a mysterious illness as a teenager, one characterized by weight loss, a capricious and occasionally voracious appetite, episodic vomiting and diarrhea, pallor, frequent faints and episodes of shortness of breath. She probably had at least one spell of amenorrhea. We know that she was physically active throughout this illness. An accomplished horsewoman and dancer, she would often hunt all day and dance in the evening. The English ambassador, Sir Francis Throckmorton, wrote home, '. . . the Scottish Queen in my opinion looked very ill on it, very pale and green, and withal short breathed, and it is whispered here among them that she cannot live long'. This illness appears to have begun when Mary was 14 and involved in a long, public and vexatious disagreement with her French governess, Mme de Parois. Mme de Parois thought her perks of office included what she could raise from the sale of Mary's used state gowns, while Mary believed the money could be put to better uses, like paying for more dresses. The matter resolved itself when Mme de Parois retired. Mary was very healthy indeed by the time she returned to Scotland as an 18-year-old Queen. The temptation to conclude (McSherry, 1985) that she had a serious eating disorder is almost irresistible.

# Other causes of excessive eating

Hyperphagia (uncontrollable appetite) may be a feature of organic medical conditions such as Prader–Willi syndrome, Kleine–Levin syndrome and hypothalamic brain tumors.

Robert Hall is a Scottish legend, celebrated in folk lore, a man who lived in the West of Scotland in the first half of the 19th century. Known as 'Rab Ha', the Glasgow Glutton', he had a insatiable appetite from birth and, as an infant, kept his distraught parents awake at night with high-pitched cries for food. As a child, he was known to steal bones and food from the family dog. Rob was so fat that he could barely get through the doorway of his home by the time he was 16 years of age. He started his working life as a farm laborer, but soon gave that up to attend hunts and horse races, as he was very fond of horses. He became famous throughout Scotland for his prodigious feats of gluttony and was the perpetual winner of eating contests between himself and other gluttons from far and wide. His opponents often ate so much they vomited, but Rab never did, he just kept on eating. He was described as having 'an unbounded voraciousness of appetite' and was never known to complain of indigestion or abdominal discomfort. He died in a hay loft in 1843. A newspaper of the time reported that he had been intoxicated and smothered in the straw. His history strongly suggests that he had Prader–Willi syndrome and that his death was due to obstructive sleep apnea secondary to his morbid obesity (Timmins and McSherry, 2000).

DSM-IV-TR includes a condition called 'binge eating disorder' within the category EDNOS, but does not classify it as a separate discreet entity. Strongly associated with mood disturbances, particularly depression, binge eating is thought to be a major factor in about 5% to 8% of persons affected by obesity, especially in its more severe forms (Marcus, 1995). Affected individuals have recurrent episodes of uncontrollable consumption of excessive quantities of food over a short period of time. Eating past satiety to the point of physical discomfort, they dissociate eating from hunger, eat rapidly and alone, and feel guilt and disgust at their own behaviors. They do not purge, fast or undertake excessive exercise. Increased appetite may be a feature of psychiatric conditions such as depression, dementia and mania, or a consequence of systemic corticosteroid therapy and use of psychotropic drugs.

# Association with mood disorders

Persons affected by eating disorders, anorexia nervosa and bulimia nervosa are often depressed and experience feelings of hopelessness, worthlessness, irritability and guilt (Cooper and Fairburn, 1986; Halmi *et al.*, 1991). They often have disturbed sleep patterns and have difficulty concentrating. They commonly feel anxious about eating when presented with food or in social situations where they perceive themselves to be under scrutiny with regard to body shape and size. Persons with anorexia nervosa are prone to suicidal thoughts, and symptoms of obsessional and compulsive type (Hsu *et al.*, 1993). Suicide is a common cause of death among persons affected by eating disorders who die of disease-related causes. Major depressive disorders are more common in persons with eating disorders than in comparable control populations, with depressive disorder being particularly associated with bulimia nervosa and the bulimic subtype of anorexia nervosa (Halmi *et al.*, 1991). Social phobia is common in persons affected by anorexia nervosa and the lifetime risk of obsessive–compulsive disorder in a person with anorexia nervosa is four times greater than normal (Halmi *et al.*, 1991).

Do people affected by an eating disorder actually have a major depressive disorder or obsessive–compulsive disorder (OCD) as core psychiatric conditions? Most likely not. The depression encountered in persons with anorexia is usually associated with the worst degrees of malnutrition and is reversed with refeeding (Cooper, 1995a). Obsessive–compulsive symptoms are accentuated by low mood, and effective OCD therapies, e.g. antidepressants, are not usually of much benefit in anorexia (Cooper, 1995a). Both depression and obsessive–compulsive symptoms in persons affected by eating disorders are probably expressions of the starvation state (Cooper, 1995a). OCD presenting for the first time in a young woman with pronounced concerns about food and eating can be confused readily with an eating disorder as the following clinical case study will show.

**Case study**

A young woman, Dawn, was referred by her family doctor for evaluation of a possible eating disorder. She had been losing weight and experiencing episodic diarrhea for about a year. She had undergone a thorough gastroenterological work-up in a major teaching hospital without evidence of pathology being found. Her menstrual cycle had ceased about six months earlier. Concerned about her health, Dawn understood that she was significantly underweight, but was unable to gain weight because her multiple food allergies had left her on a diet restricted in food type and caloric content. Her symptoms had actually begun about 14 months previously, soon after watching a television program on salmonella in poultry. Since then she had become overly concerned about cleanliness, was unable to prepare dinner for her family because of her lengthy disinfecting rituals and habitually used her foot to flush the toilet. The pattern of her bowel movements suggested a vigorous gastrocolic reflex, a normal physiological mechanism by which food ingestion stimulates bowel activity, and an irritable bowel syndrome (IBS), a condition of unknown origin in which bowel function becomes erratic without any evidence of physical disease. From her tendency to have bowel movements shortly after eating and her intermittent episodes of abdominal cramps with loose bowel movements, Dawn had concluded that she was allergic to whatever food she had eaten just before the episode started. As a result, she had gradually eliminated so many foods from her diet that she could not maintain her weight at a time of active growth. She listened carefully to an explanation of normal bowel function, accepted reassurance that she did not have food allergies and increased her food consumption cautiously over the next several weeks. Dawn gradually gained weight and, with coaching, was able to minimize her obsessive–compulsive behaviors to the point where she could now prepare the family dinner in time for her parents coming home from work.

Are eating disorders simply variant anxiety disorders? The anxiety experienced around food and in social situations by persons affected by eating disorders is readily understood within the context of the disorders themselves. The core features of heightened self-awareness, fear of fatness and fear of certain foods occur within a disordered belief system and are themselves sufficient to generate anxiety that is independent of any anxiety disorder. It is worth remembering that many persons suffering from social phobia experience profound anxiety around eating in public or in the company of others.

# Eating disorders in males

While there are no reliable prevalence figures for eating disorders in males overall, eating disorders in males are becoming a significant clinical concern. Although there are more overweight men than overweight women, overweight men seem to be less concerned with body weight and image than are overweight women. To turn an epigram, and using hyperbole to make a point, women are seen as concerned about size and weight, men are perceived to be concerned about strength and physical capacity. The numbers of men and women participating in regular exercise programs are pretty well equal, although articles and advertisements in fitness magazines aimed at a predominantly female audience tend to focus on weight (diet, calorie intake, etc.), while similar media messages aimed at men focus on shape (muscle toning, body building, weight lifting, etc.) (Andersen, 1990; Drewnoski and Yee, 1987). Given their known predilection for body mass, men are more likely than women to abuse anabolic steroids and some of their behaviors have an obsessional–compulsive quality similar to those seen in women struggling with eating disorders, a sort of reverse anorexia nervosa.

**Case study**

John, a 22-year-old male, consulted at his girlfriend's insistence. He was a part-time student who worked at a pub as a part-time bouncer and spent most of the rest of his spare time working out at a gym. He had started using anabolic steroids to help him reach his targets in muscle mass and physical strength. His girlfriend was concerned at his irritability and frequent rages, as well as the possible long-term health consequences. John actually asked for help in understanding why he needed to take steroids to increase his size and strength. He found that he continually compared himself to other men and felt compelled to be the biggest, strongest man in his circle of acquaintances. His attitudes to size and shape, though 180 degrees at variance, were reminiscent of those typical of a person with anorexia nervosa, complete with habitual use of a hazardous weight-gain measure. After several visits, he was asked, 'Why do you have to be the biggest and strongest?' He replied, 'So nobody can hurt me', and confided that he had been sexually abused by a friend of his father when he was 12 years old. Convinced that his father knew about the incident as it was occurring, he took the fact that his father did not interfere as evidence that 'you have to look out for yourself in this world, nobody's going to bother about you except you yourself!' He felt threatened and intimidated by other men whose size and build rivalled his own. He had to be in control of every situation.

Male jockeys, flight attendants, swimmers, models and dancers are vulnerable to eating disorders because of the requirements of their vocations and their use of hazardous weight-loss measures (Mickalide, 1990). Jockeys, for example, habitually use self-induced vomiting, restricted food intake, excessive exercise and prolonged use of saunas, together with laxatives, appetite suppressants and diuretics to make their weights (King and Mezey, 1987). Wrestlers at high school and college levels frequently have repeated cycles of weight gain/loss using similar means of rapid weight reduction (Perriello et al., 1995). Behaviors like these have the potential to change resting metabolic rates and place future weight control in jeopardy as well as having more immediate harmful effects like electrolyte disturbances, nutrient deficiencies and compromised physical strength and stamina.

The relationship of eating disorders in males to sexual orientation is currently the subject of debate. A population-based study of adolescents examined sexual orientation and prevalence of body dissatisfaction and eating disordered behaviors (French et al., 1996). Homosexual orientation was found to be associated with greater body dissatisfaction and problem eating behaviors in males, but less body dissatisfaction in females. A retrospective chart audit of 135 males treated for eating disorders at a tertiary care center concluded that homosexuality/bisexuality appeared to be a specific risk factor for eating disorders in males, particularly for bulimia nervosa (Carlat et al., 1997). The high rates for major depressive disorder (54% of all patients), substance abuse (37%) and personality disorder (26%) in the study population make it difficult to generalize its conclusions.

# Eating disorders and sleep

Many persons struggling with eating disorders report disturbed sleep patterns and some report night-time eating as a problem. Problematic night-time eating may be due to sleep-related eating disorders with altered alertness, binge eating disorder and bulimia nervosa with night-time eating, dissociative states and the Kleine–Levin syndrome (Shenck and Mahowald, 1994). It may also be due to night-eating syndrome (Stunkard et al., 1955), a specific condition that affects about 1.5% of the general population and perhaps as many as 27% of the morbidly obese undergoing obesity surgery (Rand et al., 1997). Night-eating syndrome is characterized by binge eating either before sleep onset or after wakening (American Sleep Disorders Association, 1990) and affected individuals typically maintain full awareness of their behaviors during and after eating binges.

Night-time eating can be a major problem for persons affected by an eating disorder where binge eating is a feature. McSherry and Ashman (1990) have postulated that individuals who restrict their appetites and food intake during the day may find themselves waking at night with eating impulses that resist their usual coping efforts. The situation of being in bed, in the dark, lying still when the house is quiet, is one of sensory deprivation. People struggling with eating disorders may find the strategies they use for appetite control under normal, daytime circumstances are now ineffective since they rely on an ability to focus on something purposeful and to distract themselves from eating impulses. The result is a nocturnal eating binge during which affected individuals may consume so many calories that they gain weight, reinforcing their fears of fatness and causing them to decrease their daytime food intake even further. The resulting vicious circle can be broken by an increase in daytime food intake (McSherry and Ashman, 1990). Sleep studies may be required to differentiate between a sleep-related eating disorder and an eating disorder-related sleep disorder.

### Case study
Anne, a 22-year-old female student, sought medical advice for 'an eating and sleeping disorder' of four months' duration. She stated that her eating habits were out of control, as was her whole life. A relationship had terminated about the time her health problems began. She had begun binge eating at first and then found herself alternately fasting and bingeing

in an effort to control her weight. She had been inducing vomiting several times daily for six or eight weeks. Her sleep pattern gradually worsened until she found herself waking at night with such intense food cravings that she could not return to sleep until they were satisfied. She kept very little food in her apartment and found herself irresistibly consuming food belonging to her room mates during nocturnal eating binges. Not surprisingly, this was causing a good deal of friction between her and her formerly supportive friends. She was preoccupied with thoughts of food, eating and body weight. Despite continued purging, her weight rose and she resorted to drastic daytime restriction of food intake as a compensatory device. This seemed to make her nocturnal eating problem worse and she had recently asked her room mates to lock her in her room overnight to keep her away from food.

She gave a history suggestive of anorexia nervosa at age 19 when she reduced her weight to 90 lbs by rigorous dieting and maintained it at that level for about a year. She was 5′ 4″ tall and a weight of 90 lbs meant that her Body Mass Index (BMI) would then have been 16. Her menstrual cycles had ceased until her weight rose to 110 lbs approximately a year later. Her weight had gradually increased to 140 lbs over the next two years, partly as a result of reduced opportunities for exercise and partly as a result of her eating binges.

Anne agreed to participate in a program of cognitive-behavioral therapy combined with insight-oriented psychotherapy after being advised that she was affected by bulimia nervosa. The physician explained that sleep disturbance is a common feature of bulimia nervosa and nocturnal waking places affected individuals in a situation of sensory deprivation where eating impulses are difficult to control, since there is limited opportunity to use techniques of distraction. Her treatment included a dietary plan that emphasized an increase in daytime calorie consumption and having low-calorie snacks available to satisfy nocturnal eating impulses. Sleep improved and nocturnal waking ceased almost immediately when her diurnal calorie intake improved. Although Anne's subsequent attendances at follow-up appointments were erratic, her daytime binge/purge episodes were greatly reduced in frequency and severity, and she was free of nocturnal eating binges when seen a year later.

# Stealing and impulse control

The question of impaired impulse control in persons struggling with eating disorders is an interesting one with curious ramifications. Stealing/shoplifting is more common in persons struggling with eating disorders than in the general population. One study (Vandereycken and Van Houdenhove, 1996) found that 47% of a group of patients meeting DSM-IV-TR criteria for anorexia nervosa and bulimia nervosa reported stealing. The proportion of stealers was highest when the diagnosis was anorexia bulimic subtype (54.8%) compared to bulimia (48.7%) and restricting anorexia (35.3%). The majority of items stolen were related to the eating disorder in some way, e.g. food, money, laxatives, diet pills, etc., and many respondents stated that it was their embarrassment at shopping for these particular items that led to their shoplifting in the first place. Is shoplifting in this situation an impulse disorder or just plain stealing? The author's experience is that persons with eating disorders will go to considerable lengths and incur great risks to obtain food when they can no longer afford to indulge their bulimic binges.

**Case study**
A female university student consulted her physician regarding symptoms of an eating disorder. She clearly had bulimia nervosa and confided that she would most likely be unavailable to participate in a treatment plan as she expected to be jailed for shoplifting the next day when she appeared in court to answer for her fourth offence. She had been in court on three previous occasions charged with the same offence, stealing food from a convenience store. She had been given a conditional discharge for her first offence, served 30 days in jail on the second charge and 60 days on the third. She now expected a nine-month sentence. Her family knew nothing of any of this as she had told them that she was traveling abroad each time she had been jailed and had given them the name of a friend and confidante as an intermediary through whom she could be contacted. She had said nothing about her eating disorder to the judges and had not been represented by a lawyer at any of her trials. She saw the indignities of her arrest, trial and imprisonment as appropriate consequences of her personal unworthiness. 'At least', she said, 'in prison it's easy to stick to regular eating habits!' At the suggestion of her physician she consulted a lawyer that day, subsequently explained the situation to the judge and was discharged on condition that she remained under her physician's care for necessary treatment. She saw this humanity on the part of the legal system as a powerful reassurance of self-worth.

# Population screening

A number of self-report questionnaires have been developed to assess the presence and severity of abnormal eating attitudes and behaviors. The Eating Attitudes Test (EAT) is a 40-question self-report questionnaire (Garner and

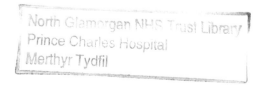

Garfinkel, 1979) that was probably the first screening device to measure the frequency and severity of symptoms common in anorexia nervosa. The Eating Attitudes Test–26 (EAT 26) is an abbreviated version (Garner *et al.*, 1982) of the EAT that estimates the likelihood of a respondent having a clinically signifi-cant eating disorder based on the frequency and severity of attitudes and beha-viors in the areas of dieting, bulimia nervosa and food preoccupation, and oral control. The Eating Disorders Inventory (EDI) (Garner *et al.*, 1983) is another widely used screening tool and the Bulimic Investigatory Test, Edinburgh (BITE) (Henderson and Freeman, 1987) is more recent and more specific to the detection of bulimia.

Although the actual diagnosis of an eating disorder can only be made at a clinical assessment, screening instruments have a demonstrated utility in iden-tifying individuals at risk for an eating disorder who should be interviewed. However, they lack the ease and simplicity that would allow useful enquiry about eating attitudes and behaviors to become part of the systems review in routine generalist clinical encounters, especially in family practice.

The SCOFF questionnaire (Morgan *et al.*, 1999) is a recent and promising development. There are five SCOFF questions.

1  Do you make yourself Sick because you feel uncomfortably full?
2  Do you worry you have lost Control over how much you eat?
3  Have you recently lost more than One stone (14 lbs) in a three-month period?
4  Do you believe yourself to be Fat when others say you are too thin?
5  Would you say that Food dominates your life?

One point is scored for every 'yes' answer. Scores of two or more are 100% sen-sitive for anorexia nervosa and bulimia nervosa, alone or in combination, with a specificity of 87.5%. Although the questionnaire's clinical usefulness has not yet been established in a primary care population, this author believes it is a highly appropriate series of non-threatening questions for the non-specialist clinician to ask in a situation where a person presents with a physical complaint or finding suggestive of an eating disorder, e.g. evaluation of weight loss or painless salivary gland swelling in an adolescent or young adult.

# Clinical presentations

Most people affected by eating disorders eventually come to the attention of a health professional one way or another. Dentists may recognize the dental con-sequences of repetitive vomiting, erosion of dental enamel (perimyolysis) and painless enlargement of the salivary glands (sialadenosis). School nurses may notice that individual students are prone to fainting spells. Physical education teachers may notice that a student's stamina and physical capacity are substandard. Team physicians and coaches may be aware of the 'female athletic triad', disordered eating, cessation of menstruation and osteoporosis, and recognize it in a female athlete. Family physicians or obstetricians may find themselves caring for a pregnant woman with a history of an eating disorder or with onset of an eating disorder during pregnancy. Physicians caring for young women with diabetes may become aware of an extra dimension of difficulty in obtaining good diabetic control, leading to recognition of the presence of an eating disorder. Guidance teachers may recognize signs of a mood disturbance in students whose academic performance is deteriorating. Affected adolescents and teenagers are often taken to their family physicians by their parents for evaluation of weight loss or failure to thrive, because their binge/purging has been observed or suspected, because of a complication of their condition such as sialadenosis or because the adolescent or teenager has shared his or her problem with a parent.

People struggling with eating disorders may consult physicians about menstrual irregularities, infertility, fatigue, reduced exercise tolerance, abdominal pain and diarrhea (even when using laxatives) and sleep disturbance. They may present with the statement that they have an eating disorder and are seeking help. They can be highly secretive about their eating behaviors and attitudes and their appearances. Young people living at home can hide their disordered eating activities and weight loss by such subterfuges as pretending to eat dinner with friends and by adopting a baggy, multilayered style of dress that camouflages their body shape.

An eating disorder can be a presenting feature of post-traumatic stress disorder (PTSD) in women (Dansky *et al.*, 1997). The clinical picture is one of pathological eating behaviors and attitudes occurring in an individual suffering from depressed mood, panic attacks and 'flashbacks', in association with avoidance behavior and heightened physiological arousal.

# Physical complications

Patients with eating disorders have two kinds of physical health problems; those caused by hazardous weight-loss measures and those caused by starvation itself. The consequences of hazardous weight-loss measure use may be fatal, whereas the results of chronic starvation are generally reversible with refeeding, improved nutrition and weight gain.

Table 1.1 lists known medical complications of eating disorders, together with their complications, causes and possible treatment strategies.

Hazardous weight-loss measures include self-induced vomiting, misuse of laxatives and diuretics, and excessive exercise. Self-induced vomiting (Goldbloom and Kennedy, 1995) can cause tears in the esophageal mucosa or inner

**Table 1.1:** The medical complications of eating disorders

| Complication | Cause | Management |
|---|---|---|
| **Metabolic** | | |
| metabolic alkalosis ± hypokalemia | vomiting<br>laxative abuse<br>diuretic abuse | stop vomiting<br>stop laxatives<br>stop diuretics<br>potassium supplements |
| hyponatremia | laxative abuse<br>diuretic abuse | stop laxatives<br>stop diuretics<br>correct starvation<br>and dehydration |
| elevated serum amylase edema | vomiting<br>starvation<br>bingeing<br>refeeding | stop vomiting<br>restore weight, fluid balance<br>stop binge/purging<br>avoid diuretics<br>ACE inhibitors may help |
| hypercholesterolemia | unknown | balanced diet |
| **Dermatological** | | |
| dry skin and nails | starvation | weight restoration<br>topical emollients |
| dyshydrotic dermatitis of hands | compulsive washing | reduce washing frequency<br>topical emollients<br>topical steroids |
| recurrent localized skin eruption | fixed drug reaction | avoid laxatives containing phenolphthalein |
| thinning scalp hair | starvation | weight restoration |
| lanugo carotenemia | starvation<br>high intake of foods containing vitamin A | weight restoration<br>harmless: reduce intake<br>squash, carrots, etc.; weight restoration |
| calluses on hands (2nd MTP joint of dominant hand) | frequently inducing vomiting | stop inducing vomiting |
| angular stomatitis | frequent vomiting | stop vomiting<br>topical steroid, antifungal, antibiotic |
| **Ear, nose and throat** | | |
| sialadenosis | binge/purge cycles | stop binge/purge cycles<br>antibiotics unnecessary |
| perimyolysis | vomiting | stop vomiting<br>consult dentist |

**Table 1.1** (*continued*)

| Complication | Cause | Management |
|---|---|---|
| recurrent laryngitis | frequent vomiting | stop vomiting<br>if involuntary – prokinetic +<br>antisecretory agents |
| **Cardiovascular** | | |
| peripheral cyanosis | starvation | weight and fluid restoration |
| bradycardia | starvation | weight and fluid restoration |
| hypotension | starvation | weight and fluid restoration |
| syncope | starvation | weight and fluid restoration |
| arrhythymias | starvation<br>hypokalemia | weight and fluid restoration<br>potassium supplements |
| cardiomyopathy | starvation<br>ipecac abuse | weight and fluid restoration<br>vitamin supplements<br>stop ipecac (emetine) abuse |
| **Gastrointestinal** | | |
| bloating/early satiety | starvation | small meals<br>prokinetic agent |
| involuntary vomiting | lower esophageal<br>sphincter incompetence<br>esophageal dismotility | antisecretory agent<br><br>prokinetic agent |
| constipation | starvation | high-fibre diet<br>stool softeners<br>avoid laxatives |
| diarrhea | laxative abuse | stop laxatives |
| hematemesis | vomiting | Mallory-Weiss tear<br>Boerhaave's syndrome (rare) |
| esophageal or gastric dilation | severe bingeing | medical emergency<br>decompression |
| pancreatitis | binges<br>starvation | therapy of pancreatitis |
| **Endocrine** | | |
| amenorrhea | low body weight<br>stress, erratic eating | weight restoration<br>cyclical estrogen and<br>progesterone |
| hypothermia | starvation | weight restoration |
| decreased T3, T4 | starvation | weight restoration |
| increased growth hormone,<br>cortisol levels | starvation | weight restoration |

(*continued*)

**Table 1.1** *(continued)*

| Complication | Cause | Management |
|---|---|---|
| breakthrough bleeding with oral contraceptive use | vomiting, laxative abuse | stop vomiting<br>stop laxatives |
| **Musculoskeletal**<br>delayed bone maturation<br>small stature | starvation | weight restoration<br>high calcium intake<br>cyclical estrogen &<br>progesterone |
| osteopenia | | |
| osteoporosis | | |
| stress fractures | starvation | as above |
| tetany | metabolic alkalosis | stop vomiting, etc.<br>correct electrolyte balance |
| **Hematological**<br>mild anemia | starvation | weight restoration |
| neutropenia | | balanced diet |
| thrombocytopenia, low | | iron supplements |
| erythrocyte sedimentation rate | | |
| **Neurological**<br>seizures | metabolic abnormality | correct abnormality |
| cortical atrophy | starvation<br>high cortisol | weight restoration |
| cognitive impairment, mood disturbance | starvation | weight restoration |

lining (Mallory–Weiss syndrome) or tears that penetrate the full thickness of the esophagus (Boerhaave's syndrome). A Mallory–Weiss mucosal tear can be suspected when attempts at self-induced vomiting produce vomitus that is stained by bright red blood. Boerhaave's syndrome is much more serious as the presence of a full-thickness esophageal tear allows stomach contents to be expelled into the chest's internal spaces during vomiting, producing a life-threatening condition requiring immediate surgical drainage and repair.

Patients with eating disorders, especially anorexia nervosa, often complain of constipation, abdominal discomfort and stomach bloating caused by demonstrable delays in gastric emptying after food and prolonged bowel transit times (Stacher *et al.*, 1992). Delayed gastric emptying may be a significant factor in maintaining abnormal eating attitudes and behaviors as the sensation of epigastric fullness may be misinterpreted by patients as confirmation of their worst fears, that food has turned to fat, and encourage them to respond inappropriately by vomiting, using laxatives or overexercising. Many patients with eating disorders consume large amounts of laxatives because they enjoy the feeling of a flat, empty stomach, although they may not like the accompanying cramps and diarrhea, and in the mistaken belief that laxatives reduce the amount of calories absorbed from food. Long-term use of laxatives tends to produce laxative dependence (the cathartic colon) (Goldbloom and Kennedy, 1995). Abrupt cessation of laxative use will result in decreased spontaneous bowel activity for some time until normal peristaltic function becomes gradually restored. In the meantime, patients affected by eating disorders will assume that their abdominal discomfort and distension are caused by rapidly increasing body fat deposition and may resume laxative use or resort to further reductions in food intake, increased frequency of vomiting or renew their exercise programs with fresh, if misguided, vigor. Stimulant laxatives containing phenolphthalein may damage the bowel's nerve supply, leading to a reduction in normal bowel peristaltic activity. Fortunately, phenolphthalein-containing laxatives have been withdrawn from the North American market, because of concerns regarding their potential as cancer-causing agents.

Some patients who have induced vomiting frequently over long periods of time find that they vomit involuntarily, especially after eating larger than usual quantities of food, or vomit on such minimal provocation as hand pressure in the epigastric area. Heartburn can be a common and distressing complaint, especially in bulimia nervosa, when the lower esophageal sphincter, the valve preventing stomach contents from flowing back into the esophagus, becomes dysfunctional. Prokinetic agents (American Psychiatric Association, 2000a) such as domperidone can help by minimizing delayed gastric emptying and/or bowel transit times. H2 blockers, e.g. cimetidine and ranitidine, or proton pump inhibitors, e.g. omeprazole or pantoprazole, may also be helpful by suppressing production of gastric acid.

Repeated vomiting, laxative-induced diarrhea and diuretic abuse, alone or in combination, all produce a metabolic acidosis with associated electrolyte abnormalities as chloride is lost in emesis, bicarbonate in stools and potassium lost in emesis, stools and urine (de Zwaan and Mitchell, 1993). Hypokalemia (low serum potassium) is associated with serious abnormalities of cardiac electrical conduction, including fatal rhythm disturbances such as ventricular fibrillation. Persons using syrup of ipecac to stimulate vomiting are at particular risk since emetine, the active ingredient in syrup of ipecac, is potentially cardiotoxic at the best of times and its potential becomes more real when the serum potassium level is below normal. Hypokalemia can also be a major consideration when persons with an eating disorder also have asthma and use bronchodilating medications, including inhalers. Bronchodilating medications are not completely selective for the airways and most, if not all, stimulate the heart to some degree. The possibility is that use of regular bronchodilating asthma medications may result in serious disturbances of heart rhythm in patients who are hypokalemic because of their vomiting and laxative or diuretic abuse. Binge eating can produce acute gastric dilatation (Mitchell, 1995), a serious problem that may require surgical decompression to avoid gastric rupture.

Many persons affected by eating disorders become acutely sensitive to fluctuations in dietary food and salt intake. Binge eating after a fast or consumption of salty foods may produce dramatic weight gain, often accompanied by visible facial swelling and other signs of generalized fluid retention (Mitchell, 1995) such as tightness of clothing, rings, watchbands, etc. To the affected person, this reinforces the superstitious belief that food has been converted instantly to fat and produces an inappropriate response that often perpetuates the problem, e.g. vomiting, excessive exercise or abuse of laxatives and diuretics. The actual explanation is purely physiological, persistent activation and heightened sensitivity of the hormone system (renin–aldosterone–angiotensin) that regulates salt and water balance. The term 'idiopathic cyclical edema' was formerly used to describe a syndrome in women characterized by recurrent fluid retention and weight gain unrelated to the menstrual cycle. Affected individuals often obtained prescriptions of diuretics, but the general observation was that diuretic use tended to become chronic and seemed only to reinforce the condition. It has since been established that the syndrome occurred mainly in women with abnormal scores on tests of eating attitudes and behaviors (Bihun et al., 1993). The syndrome has disappeared from current medical usage.

Repeated vomiting in association with binge eating may produce sialadenosis, a condition of benign enlargement of the salivary glands that may mimic mumps when the parotid glands are involved (Altshuler et al., 1990). Affected salivary glands may be beneath the chin (submental), beneath the jaw (submandibular), or just below and in front of the ears (parotid). They are painless, not tender to touch, usually symmetrical and settle spontaneously with reductions in frequency and severity of binge/purge episodes. They are not caused by infection and antibiotics are unnecessary (McSherry, 1999), as are imaging studies searching for stones or other forms of duct obstruction.

Persons affected by eating disorders where vomiting is a frequent and prominent feature often develop serious dental problems due to erosion of dental enamel, perimyolysis (Altshuler et al., 1990). The condition usually starts on the surface of the upper front teeth facing the palate, the site where regurgitated gastric acid contents tend to encounter teeth first, and may progress to involve all teeth. Dentists may be the first health professionals to identify eating disorders when they see oral health consequences typical of repetitive vomiting in their patients.

Malnourished individuals suffering anorexia nervosa before puberty may have arrested physical and sexual development, and may not ultimately reach anticipated heights (Klibanski *et al.*, 1995). Levels of luteinizing and follicle-stimulating hormones remain low. This produces a condition technically described as hypogonadotropic hypogonadism, where sex hormone levels are low because the brain fails to produce the usual triggers (neurotransmitters) for their production (Fichter, 1992). The effects are failure of normal breast development and reduced fertility in women (Stewart *et al.*, 1990), and lack of sexual interest and function in affected men. Prolonged secondary amenorrhea, cessation of menstrual periods after menstruation has been established, a requirement for anorexia nervosa diagnosis, places affected women at risk for osteopenia and osteoporosis with increased potential for pathological fractures (Rigotti *et al.*, 1991). Many women affected by bulimia nervosa have irregular menstrual cycles, thought to be the consequence of erratic gonadotropic (sex) hormone production when neurotransmitter production is impaired by inconsistent dietary intake of essential precursors.

Generalized muscle weakness and loss of muscle mass are common features in persons struggling with anorexia nervosa. Slow heart rate (bradycardia) and low blood pressure (hypotension) are common findings in starvation states (Schocken *et al.*, 1989) and put affected individuals at risk for fainting episodes and limit their exercise tolerance. The presence of carotenemia, an orange skin discoloration, is evidence that the affected individual has been consuming excess quantities of foods rich in carotene (carrots, squash, etc.) as fillers to stave off the sensation of hunger. Individuals with low body weight may display general skin dryness, peripheral cyanosis (blue discoloration of their hands, feet, ears, etc.) and edema (swelling) of their lower legs (Gupta *et al.*, 1987). Persons affected by eating disorders who stimulate vomiting by putting their fingers down their throats may display Russell's Sign, a callus or abrasion over the second metacarpal joint (knuckle) of the dominant hand due to repeated friction with the front teeth. Lanugo, a fine downy hair growth that is most obvious on the face, but also appears elsewhere on the body, is probably an adaptive attempt by the body to retain heat when the insulating effect of subcutaneous body fat is missing. It is a common finding in severely malnourished individuals, whatever the cause.

Mild anemia is common in persons with anorexia nervosa (Goldbloom and Kennedy, 1995) and may be associated with reductions in white cell counts. Iron as a nutrient is distributed fairly widely across the food spectrum, although some foods contain more iron than others, so that individuals restricting their food intake inevitably encounter iron deficiency over time. The anemia seen in anorexia nervosa is usually normochromic and normocytic, i.e. the red cells are of normal color and size when viewed under a microscope, suggesting that the chronic catabolic, wasting state is responsible for the anemia rather than lack of a single nutrient. Evidence of frank iron deficiency anemia suggests chronic blood loss, perhaps from laxative-induced bowel problems, and should be investigated in the usual manner. Despite the low white cell count, or leuco-penia, there is no evidence that the immune function is grossly disturbed.

Vomiting and laxative or diuretic abuse commonly produces chronic dehy-dration that may, when combined with hypokalemia, lower potassium, produ-cing irreversible kidney damage (Goldbloom and Kennedy, 1995). As in any condition of chronic dehydration, there is a risk of renal calculus (kidney stone) formation. Decreased kidney function, especially in concentrating capacity secondary to inappropriate vasopressin release, may result in a mild form of dia-betes insipidus.

There is a significant mortality in anorexia nervosa. Risk of death is greatest in persons with very low body weights and purging activities that produce hypokalemia with associated disturbances of cardiac rhythm (Russell, 1979). Persons with bulimia nervosa are at risk for the medical complications of hazar-dous weight-loss measures.

# Conclusion

Eating disorders are clearly serious and complex conditions where abnormal eating attitudes and behaviors result in serious consequences for the psycholo-gical and physical health of those affected. A series of biological, psychological and social factors can predispose individuals to develop eating disorders, preci-pitate their onset at times of special vulnerability and perpetuate them over time. Understanding these factors as they form the unique experience of each individual affected by an eating disorder is an essential prerequisite for effective interventions. Optimal patient care depends upon a highly collaborative multi-disciplinary clinical team in which members operate from a common platform of principles and values. Those principles and values must recognize the pri-macy of the patient/clinician relationship and the importance of an individual patient's functions, ideas, feelings and expectations, the FIFE of the patient-centered method. The following chapters share the knowledge and insights that a clinical psychologist, a nutritionist, a family physician and a family therapist bring to the application of the patient-centered method to the care of persons with eating disorders.

# References

Altshuler BD, Dechow PC, Waller DA and Hardy B (1990) An investigation of the oral pathologies occurring in bulimia nervosa. *Int J Eat Disord.* **9**: 191–9.

American Psychiatric Association (2000a) Practice guideline for the treatment of patients with eating disorders (Revision). *Am J Psychiatry (Supplement).* **157**(1): 14.

American Psychiatric Association (2000b) *Diagnostic and Statistical Manual of Mental Disorders, DSM-IV-TR.* American Psychiatric Association, Washington DC.

American Sleep Disorders Association (1990) *International Classification of Sleep Disorders: diagnostic and coding manual.* American Sleep Disorders Association, Rochester, MN.

Andersen AE (1990) Diagnosis and treatment of males with eating disorders. In: AE Andersen (ed.) *Males with Eating Disorders.* Brunner/Mazel, New York.

Bihun J, McSherry JA and Marciano D (1993) Idiopathic edema and abnormal eating attitudes/behaviors: a study of coincidence. *Int J Eat Disord.* **14**(2): 197–201.

Braun DL, Sunday SR and Halmi KA (1994) Psychiatric co-morbidity in patients with eating disorders. *Psychol Med.* **24**: 859–67.

Bulik C, Sullivan PF, Fear J and Pickering A (1997) Predictors of the development of bulimia nervosa in women with anorexia nervosa. *J Nerv Ment Dis.* **185**: 704–97.

Carlat DJ, Camargo CA and Herzog DB (1997) Eating disorders in males: a report of 135 patients. *Am J Psychiatry.* **154**(8): 1127–32.

Cooper PJ (1995a) Eating disorders and their relationship to mood and anxiety disorders. In: KD Brownell and CG Fairburn (eds) *Eating Disorders and Obesity: a comprehensive handbook.* Guilford Press, New York.

Cooper Z (1995b) Development and maintenance of eating disorders. In: KD Brownell and CG Fairburn (eds) *Eating Disorders and Obesity: a comprehensive handbook.* Guilford Press, New York.

Cooper PJ and Fairburn CG (1986) The depressive symptoms of bulimia nervosa. *Br J Psych.* **148**: 268–74.

Dansky BS, Brewerton TD, Kilpatrick DG and O'Neil PM (1997) The national women's study: relationship of victimization and post-traumatic stress disorder to bulimia nervosa. *Int J Eat Disord.* **21**: 213–28.

de Zwaan M and Mitchell JE (1993) Medical complications of anorexia nervosa and bulimia nervosa. In: AS Kaplan and PE Garfinkel (eds) *Medical Issues and the Eating Disorders: the interface.* Brunner/Mazel, New York.

Drewnoski A and Yee DK (1987) Men and body image. *Psychosom Med.* **49**: 626–34.

Fichter MM (1992) Starvation-related endocrine changes. In: KA Halmi (ed.) *Psychobiology and Treatment of Anorexia Nervosa and Bulimia Nervosa.* American Psychopathological Association, Washington, DC.

Fosson A, Knibbs J, Bryant-Waugh R and Lask B (1987) Early onset of anorexia nervosa. *Arch Dis Childhood.* **62**: 114–18.

French SA, Story M, Remafedi G, Resnick MD and Blum RW (1996) Sexual orientation and prevalence of body dissatisfaction and eating disordered behaviors: a population-based study of adolescents. *Int J Eat Disord.* **19**(2): 119–26.

Garfinkel PE, Lin E, Gehring P *et al.* (1995) Bulimia nervosa in a Canadian community sample: prevalence and comparison of subgroups. *Am J Psych.* **152**: 1052–8.

Garner DM and Garfinkel PE (1979) The Eating Attitudes Test: an index of the symptoms of anorexia nervosa. *Psychol Med.* **9**: 273–9.

Garner DM, Garfinkel PE, Schwartz D and Thompson M (1978) Cultural expectation of thinness in women. *Psychol Rep.* **47**: 483–91.

Garner DM, Olmsted MP, Bohr Y and Garfinkel PE (1982) The Eating Attitudes Test: psychometric features and clinical correlates. *Psychol Med.* **12**: 871–8.

Garner DM, Olmsted MA and Polivy J (1983) Development and validation of a multidimensional eating disorder inventory for anorexia nervosa and bulimia. *Int J Eat Disord.* **2**: 15–34.

Goldbloom DS and Kennedy SH (1995) Medical complications of anorexia nervosa. In: KD Brownell and CG Fairburn (eds) *Eating Disorders and Obesity: a comprehensive handbook.* Guilford Press, New York.

Gull W (1874) Anorexia nervosa (apepsia hysterica, anorexia hystericus). *Trans Clin Soc Lond.* 22–8.

Gupta M, Gupta A and Habermann H (1987) Dermatologic signs in anorexia nervosa and bulimia nervosa. *Arch Dermatol.* **123**: 1386–90.

Halmi KA, Eckert ED, Marchi P *et al.* (1991) Co-morbidity of psychiatric diagnoses in anorexia nervosa. *Arch Gen Psychiatry.* **48**: 712–18.

Hawley RM (1985) The outcome of anorexia nervosa in younger subjects. *Br J Psychiatry.* **146**: 657–60.

Henderson M and Freeman CPL (1987) A self-rating scale for bulimia: the 'BITE'. *Br J Psychiatry.* **150**: 18–24.

Herzog DB, Keller MB, Sacks NR, Yeh CJ and Lavoria PW (1992) Psychiatric co-morbidity in treatment-seeking anorexics and bulimics. *J Am Acad Child Adolesc Psychiatry.* **31**: 810–18.

Higgs JF, Goodyear IN and Birch J (1989) Anorexia nervosa and food avoidance emotional disorder. *Arch Dis Child.* **64**: 346–51.

Hoek HW (1991) The incidence and prevalence of anorexia nervosa and bulimia nervosa in primary care. *Psychol Med.* **21**: 455–60.

Hsu LKG (1995) Outcome of bulimia nervosa. In: KD Brownell and CG Fairburn (eds) *Eating Disorders and Obesity: a comprehensive handbook.* Guilford Press, New York.

Hsu LKG, Kaye W and Weltzin TE (1993) Are eating disorders related to obsessive compulsive disorders? *Int J Eat Disord.* **14**: 305–18.

Hunter RA and MacAlpine I (1963) *Three Hundred Years of Psychiatry 1535–1869.* Oxford University Press, Oxford, UK.

Kendler KS, MacLean C, Neale M *et al.* (1991) The genetic epidemiology of bulimia nervosa. *Am J Psychiatry.* **148**: 1627–37.

King MB and Mezey G (1987) Eating behaviour of male racing jockeys. *Psychol Med.* **17**: 249–53.

Klibanski A, Biller BM, Schoenfeld DA, Herzog DB and Saxe VC (1995) The effects of estrogen administration on trabecular bone loss in young women with anorexia nervosa. *J Clin Endocrinol Metab.* **801**: 898–904.

Lacey JH (1982) Anorexia nervosa and a bearded female saint. *BMJ.* **285**: 1816–17.

Marciano D, McSherry JA and Kraus A (1988) Abnormal eating attitudes at a Canadian university. *Can Fam Physician.* **34**: 75–9.

Marcus MD (1995) Binge eating and obesity. In: KD Brownell and CG Fairburn (eds) *Eating Disorders and Obesity; a comprehensive handbook.* Guilford Press, New York.

McSherry JA (1984) Anorexia nervosa and bulimia: the problem of the pleasing child! *Can Fam Physician.* **30**: 1633–8.

McSherry JA (1985) Was Mary Queen of Scots anorectic? *Scot Med J.* **30**: 243–5.

McSherry JA (1990) Polycystic ovary syndrome and bulimia: evidence for an occasional causal relationship. *Med Psychotherapist.* **6**(3): 10–11.

McSherry JA (1992) *Recognizing and Managing the Medical Complications of the Eating Disorders.* WONCA, Vancouver, Canada.

McSherry JA (1999) Sialadenosis and bulimia: benign swelling of the salivary glands. *News Prim Care Eat Disord Assoc Can.* **1**(2): 3–4.

McSherry JA and Ashman G (1990) Bulimia and sleep disturbance. *J Fam Pract.* **30**: 102–3.

Mickalide AD (1990) Sociocultural factors influencing weight among males. In: AE Andersen (ed.) *Males with Eating Disorders.* Brunner/Mazel Inc, New York.

Mitchell JE (1995) Medical complications of bulimia nervosa. In: KD Brownell and CG Fairburn (eds) *Eating Disorders and Obesity: a comprehensive handbook.* Guilford Press, New York.

Morgan JF, Reid F and Lacey JH (1999) The SCOFF questionnaire: assessment of a new screening tool for eating disorders. *BMJ.* **319**: 1467–8.

Morton R (1694) *Phthisiologia: or a treatise of consumptions.* Smith & Walford, London.

Parry-Jones B and Parry-Jones WL (1995) In: KD Brownell and CG Fairburn (eds) *Eating Disorders and Obesity: a comprehensive handbook.* Guilford Press, New York.

Peveler RC (1995) Eating disorders and diabetes. In: KD Brownell and CG Fairburn (eds) *Eating Disorders and Obesity: a comprehensive handbook.* Guilford Press, New York.

Periello VR, Almquist J, Conkwright D et al. (1995) *Va Med Q.* **122**(3): 179–83.

Rand CS, MacGregor AM and Stunkard AJ (1997) The night-eating syndrome in the general population and among postoperative obesity surgery patients. *Int J Eat Disord.* **22**(1): 65–9.

Rigotti NA, Neer RM, Stakes SJ, Herzog DB and Nussbaum SR (1991) The clinical course of osteoporosis in anorexia nervosa: a longitudinal study of cortical bone mass. *JAMA.* **265**: 1133–8.

Russell G (1979) Bulimia nervosa: an ominous variant of anorexia nervosa. *Psychol Med.* **9**: 429–88.

Schocken D, Holloway JD and Powers P (1989) Weight loss and the heart: effects of anorexia nervosa and starvation. *Arch In Med.* **149**: 877–81.

Shenck CH and Mahowald MW (1994) Review of nocturnal sleep-related disorders. *Int J Eat Disord.* **15**: 343–6.

Stacher G, Bergmann H, Wiesnagrotzki S *et al.* (1992) Primary anorexia nervosa: gastric emptying and antral motoractivity in 53 patients. *Int J Eat Disord.* **11**: 163–72.

Steinhausen HC (1995) The course and outcome of anorexia nervosa. In: KD Brownell and CG Fairburn (eds) *Eating Disorders and Obesity: a comprehensive handbook.* Guilford Press, New York.

Stewart DE, Robinson E, Goldbloom and Wright C (1990) Infertility and eating disorders. *J Obstet Gynecol.* **163**: 1196–9.

Stunkard AJ, Grace WJ and Wolff HG (1955) The night-eating syndrome: a pattern of food intake among certain obese patients. *Am J Med.* **19**: 78–86.

Sundgot-Borgen J (1993) Prevalence of eating disorders in elite female athletes. *Int J Sport Nutrition.* **3**: 29–40.

Timmins P and McSherry JA (2000) Rab Ha', the Glasgow glutton: a case of the Prader–Willi syndrome. *Bull R Coll Physicians Surgeons Glasgow.* **29**(2): 17–20.

Vandereycken W and Hoek HW (1992) Are eating disorders culture bound syndromes? In: KA Halmi (ed.) *Psychobiology and Treatment of Anorexia Nervosa and Bulimia.* The American Psychiatric Press, Washington DC.

Vandereycken W and Van Houdenhove V (1996) Stealing behavior in eating disorders: characteristics and associated psychopathology. *Comprehen Psychiatry.* **37**(5): 316–21.

Walters EE and Kendler KS (1995) Anorexia nervosa and anorexic-like syndromes in a population-based female twin sample. *Am J Psychiatry.* **152**: 64–71.

Welch SL and Fairburn CG (1994) Sexual abuse and bulimia nervosa: three integrated case comparisons. *Am J Psychiatry.* **151**: 402–7.

Xenophon A (1995) Cited in Parry-Jones and Parry-Jones. *History of Bulimia and Bulimia Nervosa.* In: KD Brownell and CG Fairburn (eds) *Eating Disorders and Obesity: a comprehensive handbook.* Guilford Press, New York.

# 2

# The eating disorders: anorexia nervosa and bulimia nervosa

## The multidimensional model of eating disorders

*Kathleen M Berg*

Eating disorders are dynamic and multifactorial in their etiology. The traditional infectious disease model (a unidimensional model aimed at discovering a single cause for a disease) does not provide an adequate framework for understanding and guiding the treatment of eating disorders (Andersen *et al.*, 1997). In contrast, research and clinical experience have supported a multidimensional model (Hall and Cohn, 1999; Wiseman *et al.*, 1998; Zerbe, 1993) which looks at a combination of societal, individual and family factors which play a role in the development and maintenance of anorexia nervosa and bulimia nervosa. Initially, the individual is predisposed or made vulnerable to developing an eating disorder by the presence of multiple factors (sociocultural, individual, family). Precipitating factors or stressful life events serve to trigger the eating disorder as it becomes a way of coping with trauma, change, conflict and developmental challenges. The eating disorder is then perpetuated by a combination of personal experiences (e.g. family reactions, lack of support systems, negative experiences with treatment) and the biological consequences of semi-starvation and chaotic eating. These factors magnify underlying problems and entrench the individual in the eating disorder.

This chapter addresses the multidimensional nature of eating disorders by first exploring sociocultural issues and individual predispositions, including traumatic stress and family factors. Second, screening tools and diagnostic issues are explored from a medical perspective. The medical consequences of anorexia nervosa and bulimia nervosa and corresponding physical assessments and laboratory evaluations are described. Finally, a detailed description of the kinds of nutritional assessments used at the time of diagnosis is provided.

# The sociocultural context of eating disorders

In the Western world, we live in a culture which is obsessed with thinness, perfection, control and achievement. Furthermore, our society tends to be one which denigrates emotional expression, frowns on neediness and is spiritually impoverished. Individual autonomy and independence are highly valued and many are left longing for community and human contact. Ironically, those who are the most adept at learning and conforming to the culturally prescribed standards of beauty and behavior are the ones who are at greater risk for developing an eating disorder. Violence against girls and women is rampant in the form of spousal abuse, date rape and sexual assault by strangers. These forces have tremendous impact on the lives of girls and women and play an important part in contributing to the development of eating disorders.

# Cultural ideals of beauty

As indicated in Chapter 1, the promotion of thinness as a cultural ideal of beauty has not always been present. In prehistoric times, goddess figures were full-breasted and round-bellied. An abundance of female flesh was considered desirable and became associated with fertility and sensuality. Until the 20th century, artistic representations of women celebrated their natural fleshiness with dimpled buttocks and thighs and ample bellies. In Victorian times, women referred to their fat as their 'silken layer' (Wolf, 1991), a term which celebrated their female sexuality.

With the advent of the 20th century, this positive view of body fat disappeared and was replaced by an aversion to fat and heightened weight prejudice in Western society. During the 1920s, for example, the beauty ideal shifted to the lean, flat-chested look of the 'flappers'. In the 1940s and 1950s, the curvaceous female figure, with larger breasts, small waist and wider hips was considered attractive. With the arrival of the famous fashion model Twiggy in the 1960s, however, extreme thinness became a cultural fixation in the media. It is well-documented that the trend toward an even thinner, more unrealistic shape has been perpetuated over the past three decades (Wiseman et al., 1992). This shift to a thinner beauty ideal exists alongside the fact that actual women are getting larger, probably due to better healthcare and nutrition. The resulting disparity between the ideal and the real has helped to foster the development of a multi-billion-dollar diet industry as girls and women, battling their own biologically normal weight and shape, strive to achieve the cultural ideal.

How does one define the current cultural ideal of beauty being presented to females today? Fashion magazines and mass advertising campaigns promote a body type which is extremely thin and tall (about 5' 8" or taller). Images in the media are air-brushed and optically distorted to present the 'perfect' body image; firm and flawless, long and lean. To be attractive, the woman must have no fat on her thighs, abdomen or buttocks and very little on her upper torso. Recently, perfectly defined but small muscles and larger breasts have been promoted, still on an emaciated figure. This body shape is more like that of a preadolescent boy or a Barbie doll than a normal, maturing adolescent girl or a woman.

What is it that makes females in this culture succumb to unrealistic and dangerous pressures toward thinness? To blame the presence of thin role models, weight-loss clinics and diet products alone would be too simplistic. In the author's opinion, what has most likely promoted the relentless and widespread pursuit of thinness and perfection are the 'promises' attached to and the insidious messages underlying the current ideal of beauty. Mass advertising 'promises' girls and women that low weights and svelte shapes will make them happier and healthier, more popular socially, more sexually desirable, more successful in their careers and more self-confident. A detailed analysis of the psychic impact of the media is beyond the scope of this chapter and is presented elsewhere (Kilbourne, 1994; Wolf, 1991). However, the following list of messages was compiled from the responses of women attending 'Body Image and Self-Esteem' workshops, lead by the author. Participants were asked to look at images of women in the printed media (fashion magazines, advertisements, newspapers) and identify underlying messages regarding physical shape and behavior.

- 'The only acceptable shape for the female body is thin and fit'.
- 'You have to be perfect to be beautiful – perfect skin, perfectly shaped legs, perfectly sized breasts, perfectly thin'.
- 'It's not your whole body that's important. The female body is presented in disintegrated parts. You should focus on your breasts, your buttocks, your thighs, and your hips and correct them'.
- 'The images are confusing. To be feminine these days, you should appear weak, frail and childlike on some days and tough and muscular on others'.
- 'Don't indulge in food, especially in public. It's sinful, unfeminine and grotesque'.
- 'Be still and silent to be accepted. Be controlled, especially with your body'.
- 'Women's bodies are objects of pleasure for men. Women's bodies don't really belong to them'.
- 'Being thin and beautiful gives you power socially and professionally, especially over other women'.

- 'A woman's body is to be appreciated for its outward appearance. Bodily functions and what women can do with their bodies are unimportant; even shameful'.
- 'Don't appear as if you've aged. It's ugly and a sign of failure to stay young. You'll be written off and ignored'.

These responses are representative of the messages girls and women pick up about their bodies. The cultural definition of beauty and femininity today is thin, passive, controlled and eager to please. Pipher's (1994) belief is that eating disorders are both a result of and a protest against these pressures towards thinness:

'Initially, a young woman strives to be thin and beautiful but after a time, anorexia takes on a life of its own. By her behaviour, an anorexic girl tells the world, "Look, see how thin I am, even thinner than you wanted me to be. You can't make me eat more. I am in control of my fate, even if my fate is starving"'.

Most clinicians believe that young women need to be emancipated from these absurd pressures. To do this, we have to address weight prejudice and the stigma attached to obesity in our society.

# Weight prejudice

Prejudice against obesity is widespread in our society. It is stereotypically assumed that obese people eat more, exercise less, have more psychological problems and experience greater health risks than thin people. Excess female flesh, once a symbol of fertility and abundance, is now associated with being out of control, laziness, lack of willpower, incompetence and unattractiveness. These stereotypes are used to discriminate against fat people (Steiner-Adair, 1994). If there is shame about the act of eating in our culture, there is even greater shame for looking as if you've eaten. According to Kilbourne (1994), our culture has projected its fears of being powerless and out of control onto fat people; they have become our scapegoats. Our society has become fat-phobic and the media is rife with examples of this. It is no wonder that people are vulnerable to joining the diet craze and develop an intense fear of fat. Increasingly young children are being targeted.

# Glorification of eating disorders

Eating disorders have received a great deal of publicity through magazines, newspaper articles and television appearances by noted celebrities in sport, modeling and the arts who have lived with these problems. While neither anorexia nervosa nor bulimia nervosa are glamorous, these disorders have become associated with upper social class, fame and achievement (Garner, 1997; Wolf, 1991). For vulnerable girls and women, the favorable social connotations attached to eating disorders can actually serve to encourage and perpetuate the pursuit of thinness and the obsession with perfection.

How do we avoid the unwitting glorification of these disorders? The voices of sufferers from all socioeconomic groups, educational levels, racial backgrounds and age levels need to be heard; they are the experts on the emotional, physical and social devastation of these disorders. Media attention needs to be drawn to the loss of health and attractiveness, the denial of personal achievements and the deadening of the spirit which both anorexia nervosa and bulimia nervosa can result in.

# Social prescriptions for behavior: search for an identity

Eating disorders are not just about dieting, binge/purge cycles and the pursuit of thinness. They are also about the search for an identity and a way to survive in a culture which has been described as 'dangerous, sexualized and media-saturated' (Pipher, 1994). How do girls and women search for personal authenticity in the midst of culturally prescribed rules which stifle individuality? How can they learn to negotiate intimate relationships, learn to take risks and develop self-esteem in a society which has become increasingly violent; where date rape, spousal abuse, pornography and sexual assault are prevalent? Individuals who struggle with eating disorders don't just control their weight; they have learned to control their passions, their needs and their voices to stay safe and to be accepted. In recent years, more attention is being paid to the cultural forces that impede female development (Gilligan, 1982; Pipher, 1994). Gilligan's (1982) research has shown that as girls approach puberty, they lose their vitality, their assertiveness and their sense of themselves in order to fit the socially prescribed view of the 'nice girl'. This 'nice girl' is self-silencing and self-sacrificing. She defers to the needs of others, is accommodating and does not create conflict. She keeps her negative feelings and opinions to herself. In *Reviving Ophelia: Saving the Selves of Adolescent Girls*, Mary Pipher warns us against a 'girl-poisoning culture which limits girls' development, truncates their wholeness and leaves many of them traumatized' (Pipher, 1994). We must acknowledge these societal forces to understand the cultural climate which contributes to the development of eating disorders.

# Changing roles of women

Girls are coming of age today amidst the confusion of changing societal roles. Females are encouraged to be nurturing and assertive, homemakers and career women, independent and dependent all at the same time. The 'super-woman' image suggests that women must not only have a perfectly thin body, they must also have exceptional careers, be perfect mothers and have perfect relationships. The stress of trying to do it all can be overwhelming. It leads women to feel out of control and ineffective in meeting the challenges of life and it can lead girls to be extremely wary of going out into the world. Feelings of ineffectiveness and loss of control are common themes in the lives of those with eating disorders.

# Individual predispositions

The multidimensional model acknowledges the presence of certain individual predispositions, including personality traits and early childhood experiences which play a contributory role in the development of eating disorders. Both genetic and environmental factors have been noted in the literature. For example, Strober (1997) claims that the heritability of temperament and personality type is well-documented and that certain qualities of personality are noted in patients with eating disorders with remarkable consistency. Other authors have cited specific childhood experiences, such as discrimination and ridicule resulting from a history of obesity (Zerbe, 1993), and difficulties encountered with early menarche (Fairburn et al., 1997) as high-risk factors. The identification of premorbid personality traits and individual experiences is important in promoting early detection and treatment. Drawing on both empirical evidence and clinical experience, this section explores several factors which may predispose an individual to the development of an eating disorder:

- history of obesity and dieting
- negative experience with early puberty
- low self-esteem
- personality style
- cognitive distortions
- depression.

Again, the reader is cautioned against focusing on the presence of a single factor in detecting an eating disorder. Both anorexia nervosa and bulimia nervosa consist of a cluster of symptoms and individual variation in presentation.

# History of obesity

Recent research has provided links between a history of childhood obesity, negative body image and eating disturbance. Studies have shown that women with eating disorders and body image disturbance were more likely to have experienced social rejection with regards to their appearance as children (Zerbe, 1993). Research by Thompson *et al.* (1995) indicates that children who are overweight experience more teasing and are subsequently more vulnerable to developing a negative body image, dieting behavior and binge-eating practices. Similarly, Fairburn *et al.* (1997) found that childhood obesity, parental obesity, critical comments regarding weight or shape and dieting among family members promote dieting and increase risk for developing bulimia nervosa. It appears that being overweight as a child can lead to ridicule and criticism resulting from weight prejudice. These experiences result in negative self-evaluation and feelings of rejection. In turn, subsequent dieting and weight loss lead to increased social acceptance thus reinforcing restrictive eating practices.

# Negative experiences with early puberty

A second group of factors which have been associated with higher risk for developing an eating disorder are negative experiences with early puberty (loosely defined as puberty occurring significantly before peer group). Strober (1997) maintains that puberty presents a maturational crisis for the young woman who is already prone to self-doubt, wants a life of predictable order and has little tolerance for emotionally charged experiences. In anorexia nervosa, self-starvation, which blunts affect, demonstrates rigid discipline and controls bodily changes, is discovered as a way of returning to a simpler, less chaotic time. Early menarche has also been implicated in the development of bulimia nervosa (Fairburn *et al.*, 1997). These authors reasoned that early exposure to pubertal changes in body shape (i.e. less angular, more curvaceous, increased fat deposits) may be a risk factor for dieting, a behavior which tends to predate binge eating.

Clinical experience shows that links between early menarche (onset of menstruation) and body-image disturbance are complex and varied. Some girls who develop breasts at a younger age report teasing by male peers, brothers and fathers. These comments result in embarrassment and self-consciousness; for example, patients have described binding their breasts under loose sweaters to hide their budding sexuality. In addition, many young women received no information or advice from their parents regarding their physical and sexual development. They have described feeling fearful, confused and shocked. It is not surprising that these reactions are heightened in girls who confront puberty at ages nine or 10. In our culture, the onset of menstruation as a rite of passage is rarely celebrated. The silence and secrecy shrouding this developmental stage can promote both body shame and a profound distrust of one's bodily functions.

A related source of negative experience with early puberty is the general association of the onset of menstruation with loss; of innocence, attention and freedom. Girls have reported hearing older women refer to menstruation as the 'curse'; some have overheard their mothers' worried hopes that their daughters will not be victims of the early onset of menstrual cycles. Many girls who struggle with eating disorders report a loss of attention from their fathers with the onset of puberty. Fathers who used to engage in playful wrestling and sports with their daughters begin to withdraw from these activities. Other girls, once described as 'energetic' and 'bouncy', are now admonished for being boisterous and 'unladylike' in their demeanor. One patient expressed her reaction to this experience: 'I felt like I was suddenly inferior when I started to become a woman. I wanted to be like my brothers who had more freedom and were allowed to be noisy. Also, my father still played with them. I felt like I had failed at something and I started to hate my body for betraying me.'

# Low self-esteem

Many researchers and clinicians have recognized that low self-esteem is a common precursor to the development of eating disorders (Bruch, 1973; Garner et al., 1997; Zerbe, 1993). Self-esteem may be defined as an appraisal or evaluation of one's personal worth as revealed by an individual's attitudes, feeling and perceptions (Garner et al., 1997). In those with eating disorders, low self-esteem is evidenced by feelings of helplessness, a sense of ineffectiveness or failure, a tendency to seek external validation and extreme sensitivity to criticism. In the author's experience, these individuals are prone to derogatory self-evaluation and demonstrate a high degree of self-loathing. Human worth is rated in terms of performance and acceptance from others; the notion of intrinsic self-worth holds little meaning for them. Many patients with eating disorders do not feel deserving of the good things in life, including love, success or even food.

The persistent belief that one's personality is inherently defective contributes to an underdeveloped sense of personal identity. According to Garner et al. (1997), some patients report taking on an 'anorexic identity' in order to infer self-worth. Extreme thinness is viewed as a sign of self-discipline, personal control and special status. Clinical experience shows that individuals with bulimia nervosa are also struggling to attain this 'special status' but feel that they don't have what it takes to attain it. Jasper (1993) contends that persons with eating disorders engage in unconscious 'displacement' of their self-loathing and shame onto their bodies. The body is then viewed as unlovable, defective and in need of external control and transformation. When an individual's personal identity is shaky and confused, weight can be a particularly appealing yardstick for measuring and shoring-up self-esteem. Unlike more abstract personal qualities and emotions, weight is both quantitative and observable. In addition, 'success' at weight loss accommodates cultural rules for appearance and behavior. Any difficulty in attaining this objective tends to further lower poor self-esteem.

# Personality style

In the context of eating disorders, personality style is defined as a constellation of personal traits which make someone more vulnerable to developing anorexia nervosa or bulimia nervosa. While the strength and presentation of these characteristics vary from individual to individual, researchers and clinicians alike continue to emphasize their relevance in the etiology and maintenance of eating disorders (Bruch, 1973; Casper, 1998). The four personality traits described here are: excessive needs for control, perfectionism, excessive needs for approval and emotional sensitivity.

High needs for control manifest differently in anorexia nervosa and bulimia nervosa. The clinical expression of anorexia nervosa is associated with emotional, cognitive and behavioral inhibition and rigidity and the ability to demonstrate extreme control over food intake. In contrast, patients with bulimia nervosa display greater emotional lability and difficulties with impulse control (Casper, 1998). The following case studies demonstrate these different personality profiles.

### Case study
Brenda is an 18-year-old high school senior and has a two-year history of anorexia nervosa. She prefers order and predictability in her day and has established strict rules for herself around food intake. Breakfast every day consists of one quarter cup of dry cereal, lunch is limited to a small container of yogurt, and dinner is a small salad of lettuce, green pepper and four grape tomatoes. Deviations from this diet are not allowed and suggestions to introduce new foods result in anxiety and vehement protests. Brenda is very reserved emotionally and has learned to control anger and hurt. She wills herself to smile and appear pleasant and prides herself in her ability to persevere and endure any kind of adverse situation, including starvation.

### Case study
Wendy is a 27-year-old teacher who has struggled with bulimia nervosa for nine years. During periods of high stress she has relapses with binge-eating episodes followed by self-induced vomiting. Wendy tries to cope with stress

by eating nutritious meals and exercising regularly. However, she experiences difficulty sustaining these efforts. Instead, she tries to control her appetite with smoking and has become addicted to nicotine. On most days, she skips breakfast, eats minimally at lunch and binges when she gets home from school. Recently, Wendy has been unable to control her temper in the classroom and reports feeling very frustrated with the rules and regulations of the school system. She describes herself as a 'bit of a rebel' with a low tolerance for boredom.

Perfectionistic tendencies are a central feature of both anorexia nervosa and bulimia nervosa (Hewitt et al., 1995). Those who struggle with these disorders have extremely high performance expectations and very stringent evaluative criteria, particularly for themselves. For example, any mark below 90% may be regarded as a failure in school. Similarly, an inability to achieve the top sales in one's division may be viewed as a career disaster. This perfectionism also manifests in unrealistic standards for body size and shape. Weights that were once measured in pounds may now be measured in ounces. Strict adherence to restrictive practices around food is demanded and transgressions result in despondency and self-hatred.

Striving for an image of perfection has been described as part of strong needs for the approval of others by demonstrating conformity to perceived expectations (Bruch, 1973; Hewitt et al., 1995). Individuals with eating disorders are motivated by strong needs to gain and maintain the approval of parents, peers, teachers, coaches, etc. Their dependence on others' approval can lead them to avoid novel tasks and unfamiliar surroundings because there is no assurance of excellence in performance or ability to adapt. Heightened conformity, fears of disapproval and perfectionism may act together to maintain the eating disorder, in that the individual is afraid of exposing any imperfections and is reticent to admit to any struggles in her life.

Autobiographical accounts provide intimate details of emotional sensitivity and how it can predispose an individual to the development of an eating disorder (Hornbacher, 1998; Mather, 1997). On the other hand, emotional sensitivity is an aspect of temperament that has received comparatively little attention in eating disorders literature by researchers. There is a tendency for clinicians and researchers to focus on the advanced stages of the disorder when the effects of biological starvation have set in. At this stage, patients appear emotionally blunted and distant in their relationships. In the author's experience, those who suffer from anorexia nervosa and bulimia nervosa tend to be very passionate individuals who are terrified of the intensity of their own feelings. They feel their emotions so strongly, they can't cope with them. These are the children and young adults who have a keen sense of injustice and are inordinately concerned about the welfare of animals, the environment and other people. While they have difficulty identifying and labeling their own emotions, they are often quite intuitive and adept at sensing the moods and affective needs of others. In many families, they assume personal responsibility for the emotional well-being of other family members. In friendship, they often defer to the needs of others and put their own aside.

When mothers are asked to describe their daughters as infants, some recall them as babies who cried out for attention and then thwarted efforts to hold and soothe them. As young children, they seemed hypersensitive to touch and 'emotionally wound-up'. The following case study provides an example of emotional sensitivity.

### Case study

At 14 years of age, Sharon has been struggling with anorexia nervosa for one year. She was referred for individual psychotherapy by her family physician after spending the summer in the hospital. The discharge summary described her as cool, distant and unresponsive to group therapy. One staff member described her as arrogant and self-centered. Sharon is the second oldest of four children, having an older brother aged 17 and two younger sisters aged 10 and eight. Her parents have been separated for two years. Her father is a professional man with a history of alcoholism and her mother works at a local bank. In therapy sessions, it is difficult to get Sharon to focus on her own needs and emotions. She worries that her father will be lonely and start drinking again in the absence of his wife. She is very vigilant about her mother's emotional needs and has taken on the responsibility of caring for the younger children and preparing meals. Sharon worries about her mother's stress level in trying to work full-time as a single parent. She feels very guilty about what she is 'putting her family through' with her eating disorder and describes herself as undeserving of attention. In sessions, she is pleasant and polite, and is adept at redirecting the focus of the conversation onto others. She is tense, her eyes reveal deep sorrow at times and terror at others. She never cries. Sharon excels academically and her goal is to become a veterinarian so that she can care for sick and wounded animals.

Sharon's story is a common one among individuals with eating disorders. She is so shielded and separated from herself that she can appear cold and unfeeling to those who don't really know her. Underneath, she is a very emotional, sensitive and intense girl who feels very misunderstood.

# Cognitive distortions

Cognitive distortions in eating disorders have been variously referred to as irrational ideas, dysfunctional thoughts and reasoning errors (Garner *et al.*,

1997). Beck *et al.* (1979) originally defined cognitions as automatic, habitual thoughts that operate unconsciously to influence perceptions, emotions and behavior. These thoughts are generated by existing 'cognitive schemas' defined as relatively stable thought patterns which serve to organize and interpret new information. In eating disorders, cognitive styles exist which are maladaptive in that they are the result of reasoning or processing errors (Garner *et. al.*, 1997). The reasoning errors distort experience and result in mood disturbance and symptomatic behavior. It is important to note here the difficulty in determining which cognitive distortions are present prior to the development of the eating disorder and which are induced by semi-starvation. With regards to the latter, research has shown that semi-starvation can lead to cognitive changes including impaired concentration, comprehension and judgement (Garner, 1997). Table 2.1 provides definitions of cognitive distortions which are common to eating disorders.

The first five are adapted from a paper by Garner and Bemis (1982) which describes the cognitive-behavioral approach to the treatment of anorexia nervosa. The last five are based on a study by Thompson *et al.* (1987) which investigated the heterogeneity of cognitive and behavioral symptomatology in bulimia nervosa. Two examples are given to elucidate each distortion. The first example relates to food and weight issues in particular. The second example concerns more general issues pertaining to personal identity, such as relationships, achievements, self-worth, etc. Many of these thinking styles are common in and encouraged by Western culture. Dualistic (dichotomous) thinking and the tendency to divide the world into polarized black and white categories is a common form of reducing ambiguity in life and feeling in control. Furthermore, our society tends to be futuristic and goal-directed; many people worry about their ability to predict and control the future. Finally, the diet industry provides direct training in the kinds of thinking patterns demonstrated by patients with eating disorders. Clients are taught to 'think thin', to trick their minds into believing they are not hungry and to have lists of 'legal' and 'illegal' foods.

Recently, increased attention has been paid to the 'voices of an eating disorder' (Thompson, 1996). Thompson (1996) describes the eating disorder voice as

> 'A never ending dialogue that plays inside the mind of a person suffering with an eating disorder. Those voices and the cruel words they speak are with a person from the minute they wake up, until the minute they fall asleep. They encourage their victims to continue to abuse their bodies through starvation, bingeing, purging and other dangerous methods of weight control and can bring them to the brink of death.'

Many patients with eating disorders claim that these voices were present prior to the onset of the actual eating disorder. The patients describe the eating disorder voice as an accusatory, lying trickster with the power to convince the sufferer

**Table 2.1:** Cognitive distortions in eating disorders

| Cognitive distortion | Description | Examples |
|---|---|---|
| Dichotomous thinking | The tendency to think in extreme, all-or-none terms. Experience is categorized as black or white, good or evil, success or failure | 'I feel good about myself if I eat only low-fat diet foods. I hate myself when I deviate from this plan'<br>'If I don't plan out every minute of my day, I'll go completely out of control' |
| Personalization | The tendency to overinterpret others' behavior or impersonal events as relating to the self | 'Those people are whispering – they probably are talking about my weight gain'<br>'As soon as I started talking to the group, he said he had to run and catch his bus. He probably thought I was being stupid' |
| Selective abstraction | Basing a conclusion on isolated details while ignoring contradictory or more important evidence | 'I am special only if I am the thinnest in the group'<br>'I don't deserve to be happy. I've disappointed everyone by having this relapse' |
| Overgeneralization | Deducing a rule on the basis of a single event and applying it to another dissimilar situation | 'When I ate carbohydrates, I was fat; therefore I can't eat them now or I'll become obese'<br>'I failed the exam last week. I am a worthless and disgusting person' |
| Superstitious thinking | The tendency to causally relate two unrelated events | 'If I eat a piece of cake, it will turn into stomach fat instantly'<br>'If I let myself feel positive about a good mark on a test, I'll probably fail the next one' |
| Exaggeration | The tendency to magnify and make a catastrophe of occurrences | 'If I gain any more weight, I will not be able to stand it'<br>'Well, he hasn't called me in two days. The relationship is probably over' |
| Defeatism | The idea that one does not presently have and cannot obtain the ability to control one's thoughts and behaviors | 'I'm just not the kind of person who can have once scoop of ice cream and leave it at that'<br>'I can't get better. I'll always be this way' |

(*continued*)

**Table 2.1** (*continued*)

| Cognitive distortion | Description | Examples |
|---|---|---|
| Regret | The tendency to dwell on the past as an important determiner of present events, behaviors and emotions | 'I would be happy if only I could weigh the same as I did when I was younger' 'If only I didn't quit dance lessons. Then maybe I would be good at something now' |
| Worry | The tendency to anticipate future problems regardless of current circumstances | 'I know I haven't binged for a month now but what if I go out of control at the party and eat too much?' 'What if I say something stupid and he finds out what I'm really like?' |
| Perfectionism | Excessive personal expectations of excellence. | 'Weighing two or three pounds above my target weight is just not acceptable' 'If I can't do something perfectly, it's not worth doing at all' |

that she cannot survive without it. The constant negative dialogue entrenches the individual in beliefs that she is worthless, undeserving and responsible for the hardships of others. In the author's experience this voice is common in eating disorders. However, many patients are reticent to bring up the topic themselves, fearing that they will be told they are 'crazy'. It is essential that professionals, family members and friends understand the irrational, but powerful workings of the eating disorder voice. Ignorance of this dynamic can serve to augment frustration and reduce compassion throughout the long recovery process.

# Depression

In the 1980s several investigators suggested that anorexia nervosa and bulimia nervosa were actually variants of clinical depression (Garfinkel and Kaplan, 1986; Zerbe, 1993). Although studies have revealed common features, such as mood disturbance, family history of depression, sleep disturbances and lowered libido, researchers today generally concede that eating disorders are not simply variants of affective disorders. The current thinking is that depression is a complication of anorexia nervosa and bulimia nervosa. According to Zerbe (1993), depression among patients with eating disorders can be a result of malnutrition, low self-esteem, and impaired interpersonal relationships. In bulimia nervosa, patients may also feel demoralized about their bingeing and purging behaviors. In some patients, depressed mood may predate the eating disorders. Restrictive eating practices, bingeing and purging may become coping strategies which the patient uses in an attempt to elevate her mood thus providing some momentary relief from depression.

Zerbe (1993) also acknowledges the co-morbidity of major depressive disorder and eating disorders. Situations involving dual diagnoses can pose considerable challenges for both the therapist and the sufferer, particularly with regards to sequencing of therapeutic interventions and choice of medication.

# History of traumatic experience

In recent years, a number of investigations have examined the relationships between traumatic experience and the development or maintenance of anorexia nervosa and bulimia nervosa (Dansky *et al.*, 1997; Deep *et al.* 1999). Gleaves *et al.* (1998) defined trauma as:

'A psychologically distressing event that is outside the range of usual human experience, that would be markedly distressing to anyone and that is usually experienced with intense fear, terror and/or helplessness.'

Traumatic experiences include assaults on or threats against an individual's own physical integrity (e.g. car accidents, rape, sexual abuse, physical abuse, victimization in times of war), serious threats to or the witnessing of injury/ death against loved ones, and natural disasters (earthquakes, floods, hurricanes etc.). Survivors of traumatic events may develop post-traumatic stress disorder (PTSD) (American Psychiatric Association, 1994), a complex anxiety disorder characterized by a number of symptoms including recurrent, intrusive flashbacks to the traumatic event, nightmares, visual or auditory hallucinations of an abuser, emotional numbing, recurrent obsessive thoughts, hypervigilence and oversensitivity to stimuli associated with the trauma, spontaneous weeping episodes and panic attacks. Low self-esteem, feelings of powerlessness and hopelessness, depression and interpersonal or work-related difficulties are common secondary problems (Zerbe, 1993).

Research concerning the co-occurrence of trauma and eating disorders has been controversial. In the early 1990s, review articles concluded that there was little evidence supporting the role of sexual abuse as a risk factor for the

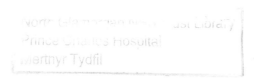

development of eating disorders (Connors and Morse, 1993). Despite this conclusion, clinicians continued to report a high incidence of sexual abuse and other trauma in the lives of girls and women suffering from eating disorders. More recently, Dansky *et al.* (1997) concluded that most researchers interpreted their results as demonstrating that sexual trauma appears to be a risk factor for the development of eating disorders rather than a direct cause. In their own study of a large, nationally representative sample of women, these investigators found that respondents with bulimia nervosa reported a significantly higher prevalence of rape, sexual molestation, aggravated assault and direct victimization (as opposed to indirect victimization such as witnessing an assault and natural disasters) when compared to individuals who did not have an eating disorder (Dansky *et al.*, 1997). In addition, the authors noted that purging behaviors were more closely associated with sexual assault than binge eating. Gleaves *et al.* (1998) found that a history of traumatic experience and post-traumatic symptomatology were common among women with eating disorders. This was especially true of individuals whose illness was severe enough to require residential treatment or hospitalization.

Links between history of sexual abuse and eating disorder subtype have also been investigated. Deep *et al.* (1999) found that the rate of sexual abuse was highest (65%) in individuals with both bulimia nervosa and substance dependence. Individuals suffering from bulimia nervosa without substance dependence had a sexual abuse rate of 37%. This rate was 23% in those with anorexia nervosa. Subjects of all eating disorder subtypes evidenced significantly higher rates of sexual abuse compared to a rate of 7% in the control group.

To date, few hypotheses have been offered to explain how traumatic experience can contribute to the development or maintenance of an eating disorder. Zerbe (1993) suggested that eating disorders may be developed as a way to dissociate from the psychic pain that accompanies memories of traumatic events. The self-starvation of anorexia nervosa sufferers rigidly focuses one's attention on food and weight and leads to emotional numbing. Bingeing and purging cycles can lead to a trance-like state which numbs out overwhelming feelings of anxiety and rage. Zerbe (1993) further claims that for those who have a history of trauma, the symptoms of anorexia nervosa and bulimia nervosa are used as a survival strategy. Food refusal, binge eating and evacuating food on demand defend against the intrusion of overwhelming feelings and provide the survivor with feelings of being in control when all controls have been taken away from her. In a discussion of the trauma re-enactment syndrome, Miller (1994) includes restrictive eating, bingeing and purging among a list of self-destructive behaviors which create the illusion of being in control of one's body. Cutting, burning, drinking and taking diet pills are also included in the list of self-injurious behaviors. Clinical experience has shown that several of these behaviors may be present in one individual. Miller's (1994) theory is that destructive acts serve several coping functions. These include: providing a sense of relief from anxiety, escaping feelings of rage or grief, producing numbness or relieving oneself from the feeling of numbness, and dissociating from the body to block out traumatic memories. Clearly, there is considerable individual variability in form and function with regards to self-destructive behavior and this must be taken into account. Two case studies are presented here to exemplify the role of traumatic stress in the development of anorexia nervosa and bulimia nervosa.

**Case study**
Heather (aged 34) was referred by her family physician for counseling following the end of her 10-year marriage. In the six months since her divorce, she experienced a drop in appetite and had lost a significant amount of weight. Her menses had ceased and she suffered from insomnia. In addition, Heather reported constant feelings of anxiety and insecurity which disturbed her greatly. On the other hand, she was happy about her weight loss and unconcerned about her physical symptoms.

Heather had been in therapy twice previously, once as an adolescent when she refused to eat and once in her mid-20s for low self-esteem and disinterest in sex. On both occasions she was put on antidepressants. The first therapist assured her parents that her behavior was just a strong reaction to a normal phase of development. The second therapist told her she was too dependent on others and needed to be more assertive.

During therapy, Heather revealed that she had been sexually abused by a male neighbor between the ages of six and nine. She had never told anyone and the abuse had been her secret for 28 years. In the beginning the abuser enticed Heather with candy and presents. When she began to protest, he threatened to kill her dog and harm her sister if she told anyone. He also convinced her that she was a 'wicked girl' and that her parents would disown her if she spoke up. The sexual abuse consisted of oral rape and fondling. As a child, Heather recalled being unable to eat her dinner on the days she visited her perpetrator. Her parents were strict and required her to sit at the table until she ate the food and subsequently vomited. When she was nine, the neighbor moved away. Heather coped by trying to be the perfect child, well-behaved, helpful and quiet. During her adolescence, she recalled having food phobias and difficulties swallowing. At the time of referral, these food phobias resurfaced and attempts to eat often resulted in gagging and nausea. Soda crackers, carrot sticks, chocolate milk and bran muffins were among the few items which Heather could tolerate. In addition to her eating difficulties, Heather had developed a strong hatred and distrust of her body. She expressed a strong desire to control both her feelings and her bodily functions.

Heather's story demonstrates the complexities in dealing with eating disorders and traumatic stress. Unfortunately, her recurrent struggles with anorexia nervosa were misdiagnosed as depression and somewhat trivialized as a phase of adolescent development and female overdependence. In addition, lack of information regarding the childhood sexual abuse made it impossible for previous therapists to link current eating problems with prior trauma. Heather's food refusal served several functions; it helped her to feel in control and dissociated from feelings of terror, guilt and rage. Because of the oral rapes, the eating of certain foods served as a trigger for traumatic memories and hence were avoided. Over the years, Heather's anxiety generalized and the list of foods to avoid lengthened. Finally, she felt special for being extremely thin. In Heather's words: 'Being this thin makes me feel like there's something I'm good at. At the same time, sometimes I feel so ashamed that I want to just disappear. It makes me feel safe.'

**Case study**

At the age of 19, Katie was in a severe car accident which resulted in permanent damage to her left hip and leg. As a pedestrian, she had been hit from behind by a drunk driver and suffered life-threatening injuries. Prior to this accident, Katie had been a very outgoing young woman who played competitive tennis and was on the school basketball team. She had been offered a tennis scholarship at a prominent university. The car accident destroyed this dream and resulted in months of hospitalization, pain and physiotherapy. During her hospitalization, Katie went through periods of deep depression. The hospital staff were reported to be tremendously helpful and encouraging during this time. Subsequent to discharge, Katie began to have recurrent nightmares about being stabbed by a stranger while asleep in her bed. She had trouble coping with stress, and decision-making tormented her. In the hospital, she had lost a considerable amount of weight; her friends admired this and told her she 'looked great'.

Katie was referred for individual psychotherapy when her mother discovered her purging (self-induced vomiting) after dinner. In therapy, she revealed that although she did not engage in planned binges, she 'overate' at meals and did not want to gain her weight back. With her lowered activity level, she was afraid she might 'get fat'. In addition, Katie was reluctant to give up the purging because it was the only thing that made her feel better. Purging relaxed her and gave her relief. Over time, she began purging three or four times a day, including meals and snacks. There was no history of eating-disordered behavior prior to the accident.

Katie's struggle with bulimia nervosa was strongly related to the physical and emotional trauma she suffered as a result of the car accident. She reported feeling that her body had been assaulted and her dreams destroyed. She experienced a loss of control over the direction of her own life. During therapy, Katie was able to access and work through the intense anger she felt toward the drunk driver who hit her. Purging had become a way of trying to obliterate her rage. It numbed out her uncomfortable feelings, many of which she was unaware or unable to name. In her mind, eating made her feel 'gross' and 'disgusting'. Having food in her stomach made her feel 'out of control' and 'spacey'. Purging distracted her from her emotions, providing a momentary calm and the illusion of being in control. Legitimizing Katie's feelings of anger, loss and fear and connecting these to the traumatic shock of the car accident became key elements in her recovery process.

# Family factors in eating disorders

*Dermot J Hurley*

Much has been written about families with eating disorders, and the significance of family patterns in the development and maintenance of these disorders. The issue of family involvement in eating disorders is important to identify, as there is an increase in the incidence of anorexia and bulimia in adolescents and young females aged 15–24 (Hoek, 1997). This increased vulnerability comes at a peak time of developmental demand for separation and individuation, causing significant problems for young persons and their families. From an individual perspective, anorexia nervosa is seen as a symptom of a deficit in the maturation of the self in the area of autonomy, self-regulation and identity (Goodsitt, 1985; Sours, 1980). Clinicians working with families with an adolescent suffering from anorexia have repeatedly emphasized the blurring of generational boundaries, excessive closeness and a tendency to avoid conflict in the family (Minuchin *et al.*, 1978; Selvini-Palazzoli and Viaro, 1988). Bulimia, on the other hand, has been linked to family-based interactional patterns characterized by hostility, neglect, open criticism, rejection and blaming (Humphrey, 1991; Johnson, 1991). Families with a bulimic member have been described as either perfectionistic, overprotective or chaotic (Root *et al.*, 1986). Bulimia is also thought to be related to profound feelings of emptiness and deficits in nurturance and empathy (Strober and Humphrey, 1987). Other studies have shown a link between blurred intergenerational boundaries in families and the development of anorexia and bulimia (Hannun and Mayer, 1984). Food refusal has been viewed as an adaptation to familial intrusiveness and overprotectiveness (Goodsitt, 1985; Humphrey, 1991; Johnson, 1991), and clinicians have repeatedly emphasized maternal overinvolvement and the failure to respond appropriately to the child's autonomous behavior (Bruch, 1978). One study looked at the involvement of both parents and found that patients with anorexia or bulimia view their fathers but not their mothers as overprotective (Calam *et al.*, 1990). Regardless of which parent is overinvolved, lack of clearly defined hierarchy in families has been repeatedly shown to be associated with an eating disorder (Minuchin *et al.*, 1978).

White (1987) sees self-denial in compliance with the dictates of the family to be the main dynamic in families with an adolescent with an eating disorder. Taking a transgenerational systems perspective, he argues that rigid and inflexible beliefs which include role prescriptions for certain daughters are transmitted from one generation to the next, resulting in the development of an eating disorder in the vulnerable individual (White, 1983).

Other family processes have been described in the literature on eating disorders. Hyper-reactivity is common in family members with bulimia, and is thought to contribute to the suppression of emotion in the affected individual (Schwartz and Grace, 1990). The bulimic family member learns not to show her feelings because of the high level of affect in other family members. Family 'imbroglio', which describes a form of transgenerational conflict involving three generations is thought to be associated with the development of anorexia in adolescents (Selvini-Palazzoli and Viaro, 1988). The 'Hyper-Americanized family' (Schwartz and Grace, 1990), which is descriptive of many high-powered, post-modern families, is considered to be a major contributing factor to the development of bulimia in young women. Notwithstanding the accumulation of clinical 'evidence', researchers still argue that there is no clear empirical evidence to support the causative role of the family in eating disorders (Campbell, 1986; Dare *et al.*, 1994). Current thinking about eating disorders proposes a multidimensional causal perspective, with biopsychosocial phenomena that result in complex interaction of many variables (Garfinkel and Garner, 1982; Strober, 1997). These variables include a specific vulnerability in the individual patient, a degree of contributory family dynamics and the assimilation of aberrant cultural messages about dieting and body image.

Some authors have suggested that it may be more relevant to question the impact of an eating disorder on the family, since there are significant effects on families in the areas of development, communication, power and control (Levine, 1996). In the case of affective disorder, it has been shown that relatives of patients with eating disorders are generally more prone to depression (Strober *et al.*, 1990). Research is still not clear on issues of cause and effect, however, and despite extensive examination of the association between family functioning and the development of an eating disorder, there are many unanswered questions about the role of family dynamics in the etiology of anorexia and bulimia. It is generally accepted that individual, predisposing family and sociocultural factors combine in some way to produce the disorder. Increasingly, the emphasis has shifted away from the family as 'the cause of the disorder', to an appreciation of the effects of eating disorders on families.

Finally, a number of studies have shown an association between eating disorders and a wide range of sociocultural factors. Various possible links have been explored including socio-economic status and gender. For example, social class has been linked to eating disorders. Fairburn and Cooper (1984) have reported a disproportionate number of eating disorders among middle- and upper-class women. Despite the relative advantages of socio-economic status and education, the subordinate role of women in society (as reflected in the family and other institutions) is thought to be a major sociocultural factor contributing to the increased incidence of eating disorders (Schwartz and Barrett, 1988).

# Family communication patterns

Although the connection between the development of an eating disorder and family interactional patterns remains elusive, a number of contributory communication patterns have been identified. Shugar and Krueger (1995), looking at communication of aggression in families with anorexia, confirmed that these families present with a strong facade of togetherness and avoid overt conflict. Le Grange *et al.* (1992) suggest that even low levels of expressed emotion (EE) in the form of critical comments from the parents of the affected anorexic adolescent are associated with continuing symptoms and are strong negative predictors of treatment in family therapy studies (Le Grange, 1999). Other researchers report less openness and more complicit avoidance among family members in eating disordered families (Kog and Vandereycken, 1985; 1989). It is reasonable to conclude that some families contribute in a direct way to the development of anorexia nervosa and bulimia nervosa by an overemphasis on appearance and achievement, by the manner in which conflict is dealt with in the family and by attitudes toward nutrition and diet. Clearly, children's views of their own growth and development are significantly affected by the way that these issues are dealt with in the family. Clinical observations show that other families contribute indirectly towards the maintenance of eating problems by utilizing solutions that exacerbate the problem, such as food surveillance and preoccupation with a patient's weight by other family members. Some families report power struggles over food beginning in infancy and escalating throughout the developmental stages of childhood. The persistence of these interactional patterns is a continuing challenge for clinicians and researchers.

It can be argued that the term 'Anoretic/Bulimic Family' is pejorative, since it implies that there are clear pathological processes that distinguish these families from 'normal' families. Though properties such as 'enmeshment' 'overprotectiveness', 'rigidity' and 'conflict avoidance' (Minuchin *et al.*, 1978) have been repeatedly identified by clinicians looking for evidence of family pathology in families affected by bulimia nervosa and anorexia nervosa, they have not been empirically validated in the etiology of eating disorders. These processes, however, do seem to play an important role in the maintenance of eating disorders. For example, in a family with an anorexic teenager, conflict between the parents may be detoured through the symptomatic child, who is inducted into a cross-generational alliance with one parent against the other which may exacerbate her symptoms and solidify the problem. The focus of pathology from this perspective is not the individual, but the structure of the family, specifically the lack of a clearly defined hierarchy and the blurring of intergenerational boundaries (Minuchin *et al.*, 1978). For clinicians utilizing this framework to understand eating disordered families, treatment is directed toward changing those patterns which have triggered the eating problem, and which contribute towards the maintenance of symptoms.

# Blaming and stigmatizing the family

Families with an individual with an eating disorder often report feeling stigmatized and blamed by health professionals, who pathologize the family and increase their burden of suffering. It is a process of misattribution, in which health professionals, observing dysfunctional family patterns, ascribe to the family a direct causal role in the etiology of the disorder. Dare and his colleagues (1994; 1997) at the Maudsley Hospital in London, UK, who have studied these families extensively, report that there is no evidence for such a causal link. The problem of misattribution is not new to the field of family psychotherapy and is similar in many respects to the 'epistemological error' that occurred in the early research in the 1960s on the role of family dynamics in the origin of schizophrenia. Concepts such as 'the schizophrenogenic mother'* gave clinical credibility to theoretical speculations about families and how they functioned without any empirical evidence to support these ideas. In confusing cause and effect, such concepts contributed to family scapegoating and to the development of interventions that were not experienced by the family as empathic or helpful. A more collaborative therapeutic relationship is encouraged with families who are coping with an eating-disordered individual. The outcome of treatment is dependent, to a large extent, on the degree to which the clinician succeeds in engaging the client and family in the treatment process.

---

*Fromm–Reichmann's term for aggressive, domineering mothers thought to precipitate schizophrenia in their offspring. In: F Fromm–Reichmann *Principles of Intensive Psychotherapy*. University of Chicago Press, 1950, Chicago.

# Family commonalities

Families living with an eating-disordered individual share many features, and have much in common, with other families in which life threatening illness is a part of daily life. There are, however, some unique features to families living with anorexia nervosa or bulimia nervosa, particularly when the patient is a child or adolescent. Despite its secretiveness anorexia nervosa is a highly visible disorder, whose effect is deeply disruptive of family functioning. Eating disorders are expressed primarily in a family context and impact directly on the patterns of family life and the rituals that organize family living. Family space is a key issue in eating disorders, as so much disruption occurs in common living areas such as the kitchen and bathroom. Frequently, the person experiencing the eating disorder is unaware of the profound impact their eating behavior is having on the family, and misinterprets the family's reaction to their behavior as an attempt to control them, or punish them for disrupting the family. Shared physical space is often where problems are most identified by families, and is a striking metaphor for the lack of psychological space experienced by family members living with an eating disorder. For example, the refrigerator (with its connotation of sustenance/nurture) may become a battle ground in which a desperate struggle for control is played out daily, with significant consequences for all family members.

Some families go to extreme lengths in trying to control the consumption or wastage of food such as padlocking the fridge, or removing all food items from kitchen cupboards. Family conflict is often most intense around food preparation, storage and general kitchen hygiene, and the family's standards in this regard may be significantly eroded by the often desperate and driven behavior toward food that is common in eating disorders. The person suffering with anorexia, in particular, is simultaneously fascinated with and revolted by food, and his or her behavior in the kitchen reflects both sides of this debilitating dilemma. Food obsessions can preoccupy the affected adolescent for hours each day, taking precedence over all other activities in her or his life.

# Some specific commonalities in families with anorexia/bulimia

While families with an eating disorder are representative of a wide range of families in treatment, there are common features shared by families who present with anorexia nervosa or bulimia nervosa as the primary problem.

- Families have very high levels of distress and concern for the individual affected by the disorder.

- Families become organized around the symptoms. Their lives may become regulated by the disorder.
- Families feel powerless and ineffective in helping the person suffering with anorexia or bulimia.
- Families show a high level of emotional reactivity toward the individual with an eating disorder. They may become overinvolved with the problem or emotionally detached from the problem.
- Emotional contagion is common in family members exposed to the disorder. Other family members may begin to experience similar feelings as the affected individual.
- Family members are 'inducted' by the symptom into problem-maintaining patterns to which they may be oblivious (e.g. checking the garbage after each meal or when the affected individual has finished eating).
- Family members are strongly reactive to the vicissitudes of this disorder in their lives; for example, the loss or gain of a small amount of weight by a person with anorexia can trigger feelings of depression or unrealistic hope in family members.

The idea that illness may come to regulate family life in unique ways, and has an organizing impact on families, is a useful concept to utilize in working with these families. Many authors have commented on the extent to which chronic illness, in particular, structures family relationships (Campbell, 1986). However, to say that the family becomes 'regulated' over time by these disorders may represent an overly simplistic or exaggerated view of how these disorders develop and are maintained. Families may appear to be completely overwhelmed by the disorder, but continue to function at a high level of competence in other areas of their lives. It is important to keep in mind when working with these families that individual vulnerability, sociocultural factors and familial influences all contribute to the development and maintenance of these disorders.

In summary, families that are at risk for the development of an eating disorder in one of their members have been identified, both in the literature and in clinical settings, by some of the following characteristics.

- Higher socio-economic families who place a premium on personal achievement.
- Performance-oriented families that value athletic/physical performance and competition with a tendency towards perfectionism.
- Parents who deny their own needs but devote an inordinate amount of time and energy to facilitating their children's activities.
- Parents who communicate messages to their children about adequacy and inadequacy based on body image, performance and the pursuit of excellence.

- Families with higher than average concerns about health and nutrition and who are preoccupied with low-fat foods and dieting.

Other family characteristics may include:

- a life-long dieting parent who communicates dissatisfaction with his or her own body, and is particularly adept at transmitting the sociocultural myth about the ideal body image
- families in which the family of origin has unresolved conflicts transferred from one generation to the next, particularly in the area of nurture, adequacy and ambition
- parents who act as powerful transmitters of sociocultural messages that deliberately target the self-esteem of young women, making them feel insecure and inadequate in their own bodies
- a parent with an addiction problem who models 'excess' or 'self-denial' as a requirement of daily living
- families in which the ritual of food, i.e. buying, preparing, serving and eating are highly charged emotional events
- families where conflict is denied or avoided, but experienced by the children as unresolved family tension, particularly between the parents
- families with a 'problem child', who is seen to be causing emotional distress for the parents. The 'perfect child syndrome' may develop, as a compensation for the disappointment or ignominy caused by the 'bad child'.

These disorders trigger bizarre and unique attempts by young persons to establish a degree of autonomy and control through food in an effort to maintain some sense of personhood and self-efficacy (Goodsitt, 1985). The family therapist must avoid the temptation to conceptualize the family difficulties solely in terms of power and control issues, which serve only to perpetuate the struggle over food and weight. Other more fundamental family issues may be submerged by the sheer weight of concern and preoccupation with the eating disorder and its effects. Eating disorders are very difficult to ignore. Despite many parents' best efforts to let the young persons take charge of their own lives, they are inexorably drawn into the emotional struggle, becoming at times as preoccupied and obsessed about food and weight as the person experiencing the disorder. Depending on the age of the young person suffering from an eating disorder, the role of the family is considered to be a critical determinant of the outcome in the recovery process. For children under 19 years of age living at home, family therapy is the treatment of choice. For individuals over 19 living outside the home, the primary recommendation is individual therapy (Dare and Eisler, 1997).

# Family patterns in eating disorders

An appreciation of the oppressive and unrelenting nature of eating disorders is essential for clinicians working with young persons and their families. The repetitive nature of the symptoms of anorexia and bulimia nervosa involved the patients and families in a cyclical pattern of self-defeating behaviors. The more the parents attempt to control the symptoms the more the young person resists parental control. This leads to an escalating cycle of conflict and resistance, leaving both sides feeling powerless and defeated (Haley, 1980).

Some authors report little general conflict in these families, but an inordinate amount of 'eating-related conflict', suggesting that food is an acceptable way to fight (Robin *et al.*, 1994). To young persons with an eating disorder, it seems that the very core of their selves is being attacked and they vigorously defend their autonomy by resistance. The parents on the other hand may be desperately trying to get their child to eat, and intrude into the life of their child in ways that would only be appropriate with a much younger child. If the parents withdraw entirely from any involvement with the problem, the young person may feel abandoned. This can trigger more depression and disordered eating. Issues of enmeshment and autonomy become hopelessly confused as each perceives the other to be the main cause of their distress. The following case study outlines a typical scenario from a family's description of living with an eating disorder.

### Case study
Sixteen-year-old Sally has anorexia nervosa, bulimic subtype.

### Scene 1:   Kitchen (7pm–8pm)
Her parents have been trying to get Sally (through a combination of appeals and warnings) to eat something on her plate for the past hour. They are now at the pleading stage. 'Just try one little bit.' Sally yields and begins to eat under duress. Her parents back off and peace is momentarily restored. Sally begins to experience early satiety and slow gastric emptying, which results in a premature feeling of fullness and discomfort with eating. She begins to panic at the fear of gaining weight and hurriedly leaves the room. Parental anxiety soars and they become even more preoccupied with Sally's problem.

### Scene 2:   Basement (8pm–10pm)
Sally engages in an intense exercise routine, becoming increasingly agitated at the thought of 'all that yucky food' inside of her. Parental agitation escalates as they listen to the noise generated by the exercise machine, resulting in feelings of anger and powerlessness. They attempt to intervene once again and their comments are perceived by Sally as critical. An argument ensues to the point of a major blow up and the parents exit, prophesying

dire medical consequences for Sally's lack of eating. Sally is emotionally distraught and runs to the bathroom where she vomits what little she has eaten.

**Scene 3:   Kitchen (midnight)**
Her parents retire to bed, emotionally exhausted after (yet again) struggling with their feelings of how this situation developed, and what they have done to contribute to this sorry state of affairs in the family. Sally begins a lonely vigil by the fridge, feeling guilty and remorseful for the hurt she is causing the family. She begins to eat in a hypnotic fashion, unaware of the amount or even the taste of the food. She doesn't correctly identify the signals of satiety and is disgusted at herself. She becomes obsessed with her discomfort and preoccupied with thoughts of food. She tries to block out these thoughts by returning to her room to read. She finds she can't concentrate and tries to sleep. Instead she lies awake worrying. She knows she'll be exhausted in the morning but she's determined to start again and get this food problem under control. The parents also report a sleepless night.

From the above example, it is clear the family is deeply involved in eating disordered behavior. They may play a central role in maintaining the disorder by engaging in patterns of interaction that perpetuate eating disorders; the contribution of the family to the development and maintenance of the disorder is a key point of the assessment process and will be explored further in Chapter 6.

# Medical assessment

*James A McSherry*

# Initial medical assessment

Anorexia nervosa is the most frequent cause of serious weight loss in North American female adolescents and should head the list of possible diagnoses when young women and female adolescents either seek or are brought for medical assessment. Causes of weight loss can be broadly catergorized as:

- conditions that result in excessive energy utilization, e.g. thyroid overactivity
- conditions that result in inadequate energy intake, e.g. cancer, systemic disease

- conditions that result in energy loss via kidneys or bowel, e.g. diabetes mellitus, Crohn's disease or ulcerative colitis
- conditions that decrease energy absorption, e.g. bowel malabsorption syndromes.

A number of comparatively rare conditions caused by genetic abnormalities are associated with hyperphagia (excessive appetite), but they are typically not associated with binge-eating episodes and are certainly not associated with vomiting. They include the Prader–Willi (Cassidy, 1997) and Klein–Levin (Gupta *et al.*, 1996) syndromes where affected persons consume large amounts of food, but lack the sense of loss of control that typifies the person struggling with an eating disorder such as bulimia nervosa.

Medical assessment begins with a medical history, and a convenient, brief screening tool, the SCOFF questionnaire (Morgan *et al.*, 1999), can be used to open the subject of eating, weight loss, purging and weight preoccupation during the standard functional enquiry if patients have not brought the subject up themselves. Every 'yes' answer scores one point and a score of two or more strongly suggests a diagnosis of anorexia or bulimia.

1 Do you make yourself Sick because you make yourself uncomfortably full?
2 Do you worry you have lost Control over how much you eat?
3 Have you recently lost more than One stone (14 pounds) in a three-month period?
4 Do you believe yourself to be Fat when others say you are too thin?
5 Would you say that Food dominates your life?

Patients suspected of having an eating disorder should be asked more detailed questions about abnormal eating behaviors, as the frequency and severity of these behaviors is directly related to the likelihood of physical and/or laboratory abnormalities being found (*see* Chapter 1). Weight and general health before the weight loss began, speed and amount of weight loss, frequency and severity of eating binges, and type, frequency and severity of purging behaviors are all important determinants of the individual patient's physical condition. Vomiting, abuse of thyroid medications and inappropriate use of laxatives, enemas, diuretics or ipecac increase the probability of the physician finding the physical or laboratory stigmata of physiological disturbances. Purging, when frequent or long-standing, can cause severe heartburn as the lower esophageal sphincter becomes incompetent, no longer able to prevent spontaneous return of acid gastric contents into the lower esophagus (GERD: gastroesophageal reflux disease). A general systems review should obviously be part of the physical examination.

When an eating disorder is diagnosed or suspected, physical examination (American Psychiatric Association, 2000) should pay particular attention to:

- height and weight, calculation of BMI (Body Mass Index) in adults (not useful in children and adolescents; pediatric growth charts are more accurate) (Kaplan, 1993)
- skin rash (possible fixed drug eruption from phenolphthalein-containing laxative abuse)
- sexual development
- presence or absence of dehydration
- enlarged salivary glands (sialadenosis)
- lanugo (fine body and facial hair growth)
- Russell's sign (scarring over the knuckles)
- acrocyanosis (blue discoloration of ears, nose, hands and feet)
- dental status for evidence of tooth enamel erosion
- cardiac status (blood pressure, heart rate, heart rhythm)
- other physical abnormalities.

Each abnormal behavior, symptom and finding must be explained to the patient in a matter-of-fact way and specifically related to problematic behaviors.

# Laboratory tests

Laboratory investigations should be as indicated by a patient's condition and presenting complaints, if an eating disorder has not yet been diagnosed. Some abnormalities, e.g. unexplained hypokalemia (low potassium) should point the examining physician in the direction of an eating disorder as a possible diagnosis if one is not already suspected. The basic laboratory assessment (American Psychiatric Association, 2000) of a patient thought to have an eating disorder should include:

- complete blood count
- electrolytes (sodium, potassium, chloride)
- kidney function tests: blood urea nitrogen (BUN), creatinine
- sensitive thyroid stimulating hormone (sTSH); to exclude thyroid disease as cause of patient's condition
- electrocardiogram (ECG); to detect evidence of low potassium or cardiac electrical conduction abnormalities.

Other investigations may be indicated when patients are severely malnourished, if the condition is of long standing, i.e. markedly underweight for more than six months or, in females between puberty and menopause, if menstruation has been absent for over a year. Other clinically useful investigations include:

- calcium
- magnesium
- phosphorus
- liver function tests
- bone density testing; to detect osteoporosis.

Other laboratory tests that may be contributory to evaluation of the person struggling with an eating disorder may be performed as part of an assessment of the presenting complaint when the presence of an eating disorder has not been established. These tests include:

- serum amylase; for evaluation of repeated vomiting
- serum luteinizing and follicle stimulating hormones (LH and FSH) for evaluation of women of normal weight who develop amenorrhea.

As with physical examination, abnormal test results should be interpreted in a matter-of-fact way as the inevitable outcome of a problematic behavior, e.g. low blood potassium as a result of purging, anemia as a result of long-standing food intake restriction, and the risks explained.

# Initial psychiatric assessment

Ideally, the initial psychiatric assessment will be carried out in a timely fashion by a psychiatrist familiar with eating disorders. That may not always be possible and the family physician may have to assume responsibility for at least a preliminary assessment of the affected person's mental status, general and specific to the eating disorder. Some family physicians with particular expertise in eating disorders may undertake this task themselves. As always, the therapeutic alliance between a patient with an eating disorder and those providing care is crucial. The gender of the care provider may be of critical importance (Katzman and Waller, 1998; Waller and Katzman, 1997) if the affected person has been abused, mentally, physically or sexually, and may have important implications for medical examinations, particularly those that include gynecological assessments.

Persons struggling with anorexia have a fundamental fear of weight gain and becoming fat that effectively prejudices their interactions with health professionals. This fear must be acknowledged as early as possible in the therapeutic relationship and an understanding reached about the goals of therapy, preferably framed in such non-threatening terms as 'becoming healthier', or dealing with specific problems.

The assessment (American Psychiatric Association, 2000) should include a full account of the patient's eating disorder symptoms and behaviors, their duration and their fluctuations in severity over time. The patient's perceptions are of fundamental importance. Understanding the patient's view of when, how and why the problem began and continues is critical to understanding the meaning and purpose that the disorder has to the patient. Patients who do not volunteer information about purging behaviors, including laxative, diuretic or syrup of ipecac use should be specifically asked. The symptoms of eating disorder frequently fluctuate in frequency and severity over time and this periodicity is an important part of the history. Present weight, highest and lowest adult weights and for how long and by what means they have been maintained are important pieces of information.

Specific enquiries should be made about substance abuse and dependency, together with symptoms of depression, anxiety and OCD. Enquiry should be made about shoplifting, suicide attempts, self-mutilation and other evidence of poor impulse control.

The family history should not be neglected. The family's attitude to the patient and the disorder – as far as the patient's perceptions go – should be explored, as should the family's history of psychiatric disorders, eating disorders and attitudes to obesity, health, exercise, achievement and appearance.

As noted previously in this chapter, PTSD is relatively common in women struggling with bulimia. One study (Dansky *et al.*, 1997) found a 37% lifetime rate, much higher than in control populations. Histories of trauma, including physical, mental and sexual abuse are therefore important and may direct the course and form of treatment.

It may be necessary for the attending physician to invoke jurisdiction-specific compulsory powers for involuntary admission and psychiatric assessment when patients are judged to be seriously at risk for suicide or death from starvation.

# Nutritional assessment

*Nancy E Strange*

Nutritional assessment of an individual with an eating disorder may be done by a dietitian at the request of the physician after the diagnosis of anorexia nervosa or bulimia nervosa, or it may be done as part of the diagnostic process.

The assessment may consist of all or some of the procedures discussed here. All of the components that may make up the nutritional assessment will be covered, not necessarily in order of importance, as that will vary from patient to patient.

The information relevant to nutritional assessment includes:

- diet history, current and premorbid, including exercise history
- weight-change history, including growth history in adolescents
- current height and weight
- anthropometric measures
- subjective global assessment
- assessment of pertinent lab values
- calculation of ideal weight, target or 'safe' weight range, activity weight, ambulatory weight and critical weight.

---

**Box 2.1:** *Nutritional assessment processes*

- Diet history, current and premorbid, including exercise history
- Weight-change history, including growth history in adolescents
- Current height and weight
- Anthropometric measures
- Subjective global assessment
- Assessment of pertinent lab values
- Calculation of pertinent weights for the recovery process

---

# Diet history

In obtaining diet history information from an individual suffering from an eating disorder, it is useful to get a 24-hour recall, and a food frequency list in addition to a detailed three- (or more) day food record. By doing this, the dietitian is able to gather appropriate information to assess the percentage of macro and micronutrient needs being met. The dietitian will also be obtaining information about the patient's attitudes about food and nutritional beliefs. It is of the utmost importance that the dietitian be completely non-judgmental in her or his collection of diet history information in order to ensure the patient's comfort in giving the information. Patients are also much more likely to be honest in giving this data if they don't feel they are is being judged. It is often helpful to 'walk' the patient through a 'typical day' step by step, starting with the first time that any food or liquid is consumed, and continue through until bedtime. When doing a diet history with an individual suffering from an eating disorder, it is often easier to get the required information if you don't refer to meal times, i.e. breakfast, lunch and dinner. Important pieces of information may be missed if the dietitian attempts to do a diet history in a conventional fashion as individuals with eating disorders often do not eat meals; rather, they tend to graze throughout the day.

It is very useful to have a 24-hour recall from a time prior to the onset of the eating disorder. This allows comparison of current nutrient intake to 'normal' nutrient intake. It also gives a glimpse into previous feelings about food and eating and any relevant issues. Sometimes it is impossible to get a premorbid diet history, simply because the patient is too unwell, and too involved in current problems with food to be able to remember how she or he 'used to eat' before the onset of the eating disorder.

A food frequency list, i.e. a list of how often the patient consumes certain foods per week or per month, not only helps in determining the percentage of nutritional needs being met, it also gives insight into attitudes about foods.

A detailed three-day food record, if obtainable, is by far the most accurate way to assess food intake. Here, the individual is asked to keep track of everything eaten and drunk for a three-day period. Whichever method is used, the dietitian then must take the gathered data and calculate the total protein, fat, carbohydrate and energy. It is also important to look at certain micronutrients, i.e. iron, calcium and vitamins A, B complex, C and D. The values of these nutrients should be compared to the Recommended Daily Nutrient Intake (RNI for Canadians, Recommended Daily Allowance (RDA) for Americans). It is then possible to calculate the percentage of the individual's estimated daily nutrient needs that are being met. Volume of fluid intake is also a crucial aspect of the diet history. It is not uncommon for persons suffering from eating disorders to be quite restrictive in their fluid intake. Dehydration is frequently seen as part of the picture of malnutrition. For example, Pam, aged 13, had, according to her mother, a lifelong history of poor fluid intake. Her mother recalled that from the age of two years, Pam showed a distaste for drinking liquids, and her mother had to think of ways of including fluid-containing foods in her daily diet. Many individuals with eating disorders will say that drinking liquids makes them feel bloated. An appropriate level of hydration is necessary in order to get accurate blood work results.

The diet history cannot be considered complete without assessing the exercise patterns. There have been cases where the individual has exercised so relentlessly that it would be impossible to maintain a healthy weight even with reasonably normal eating patterns. The following case study demonstrates that phenomenon.

### Case study

Tammy was a 14-year-old who had been diagnosed as having anorexia nervosa. She had been to see a dietitian for nutrition counselling and was eating three balanced meals and two snacks daily. The energy intake of approximately 2200 calories should have allowed her to at least maintain a healthy weight. However, her 'typical day' consisted of walking to and from school, 20 minutes each way, practising her dance routines (she took ballet, tap and jazz classes every Saturday) for an hour after school, taking the dog for a 30-minute jog after supper, and finally doing an hour of calisthenics before going to bed. This girl was five feet tall and her vigorous workouts kept her weight at 70 lbs. Obviously her 'estimated' nutritional needs were considerably higher than normal for her age and height. The activity factor played a major role in calculating her nutritional needs.

# Weight-change history

The history of weight change is an essential component of the diagnostic criteria for anorexia nervosa. The process is viewed differently for patients who have reached physical maturity than it is for individuals who are under 18 years of age. When assessing weight-change history for an adult patient one should compare current or 'minimal' weight with the individual's normal or 'usual' weight. The dietitian can thereby calculate the percentage of body weight lost. Percentage of body weight lost is calculated as the difference between usual and minimal weight, divided by usual weight and multiplied by 100.

$$\% \text{ body weight loss} = \frac{\text{usual weight} - \text{minimal weight}}{\text{usual weight}} \times 100$$

If the patient's usual weight differs significantly (more than 10%) from ideal, it is useful to calculate the percentage of ideal weight the patient is currently at. Calculation of ideal weight will be discussed subsequently in this section.

A patient under 18 years of age would be assessed differently for weight-change history. In this case, predicted weight for height and age is used. National Center for Health Statistics (NCHS) growth charts are useful in performing the measurement. Predicted weight can be obtained by evaluating past growth records to ascertain the premorbid weight-for-height percentile (Miller Kovach, 1982) by projection to the current age in the same percentile. Percentage of predicted body weight is calculated as present weight divided by predicted weight multiplied by 100.

$$\% \text{ of predicted body weight} = \frac{\text{present weight}}{\text{predicted weight}} \times 100$$

It would be a disservice to the young patient with an eating disorder to simply calculate ideal weight for age and height using growth percentiles due to the significant growth retardation or 'stunting' that may occur as a result of inadequate nutritional intake. A typical case study follows.

**Case study**
Fourteen-year-old Judy with a two-year history of anorexia nervosa was referred for nutritional assessment. At that time, her weight was 33 kg (<5%) and her height was 148 cm (5%). If one were to simply calculate ideal weight for current height using NCHS growth percentiles, the resulting weight would be 37 kg. However, by calculating predicted ideal weight using past growth records, the resulting predicted weight would be 46 kg, which is a weight much more likely to promote 'catch-up' growth for this patient, whose past growth records showed that prior to her eating disorder she had been growing at just about the 25th percentile.

When assessing weight-change history for both patients under 18 years of age and adults, the rate at which this weight changed is very significant. A large weight loss over a short period of time represents a bigger stress to the body than the same loss which has taken place more slowly.

# Current height and weight measurements

Height assessment is necessary in order to gauge ideal body weight and it also helps in determining the presence and degree of linear growth-stunting which may be seen in anorexia nervosa. Height measurement should be obtained directly at the time of assessment, using a reliable stadiometer. It should never be procured subjectively from the patient. If the patient is under 18 years of age, it is appropriate to plot this height on NCHS growth charts. It is also essential in the case of young patients under 18 to have access to previous growth records for comparison.

Weight measurement should also be done directly at the time of assessment using an accurate balance beam scale. Ideally, this weight should be done with the patient clad only in a hospital gown. Sometimes this is not possible in the dietitian's office on an outpatient basis. However, it is important for the patient to remove her shoes, and any extra layers of clothing. Patients with anorexia nervosa have been known to arrive wearing several layers of clothing with small weighted objects concealed amid the layers in order to distort the weight obtained. It is important not to obtain body weight subjectively from the patient. It is the author's experience that an individual with anorexia nervosa may overestimate her weight, while a person suffering from bulimia nervosa may underestimate her weight.

# Anthropometric measures

Triceps skinfold measurement may be used as an indirect indicator of body fatness (Miller Kovach, 1982), and therefore non-protein energy reserves. Accurate skinfold calipers (i.e. Harpendon) should be used to measure a double layer of skin and subcutaneous fat over the triceps at the midpoint of the upper arm. The reference standards and procedure described by Frisancho (1974) may be used. The patient should be standing with the arm hanging relaxed. The distance between the olecranon and acromial processes (elbow and shoulder) is measured and the midpoint marked. At the back of the arm a full fatfold is grasped between thumb and forefinger at the marked midpoint, and lifted away from the underlying muscle tissue. The calipers are applied to the fatfold about 1 cm below the fingers. The calipers must be at right angles to the arm and with the meter facing directly upwards. Once the meter is balanced the fatfold measurement is read from it. The procedure should be repeated three times and the readings averaged to obtain the final value. This value should be assessed by comparison with appropriate percentiles for triceps skinfold measures (Krug-Wispe, 1993)

Measurement of arm muscle will provide an estimate of lean body mass or somatic protein compartment. Again, the reference standards and procedure described by Frisancho (1974) may be used. The arm circumference measurement is obtained using a non-stretchable tape measure and wrapping it around the arm at the marked midpoint. The measurement is taken three times and the average of the three is used as the final value. The arm muscle circumference is then calculated as follows: arm circumference (cm) minus triceps skinfold (mm) $\times 0.314$.

Appropriate percentile charts for arm muscle circumference are also available in the *Nutritional Care Manual* (Mills, 1989).

# Subjective global assessment

Subjective global assessment (SGA) is a valid and reproducible clinical technique described and developed by Detsky *et al.* (1987).

Five features of the history are obtained from the patient. The first feature is weight change, both total weight loss in the last six months and weight changes in the past two weeks. Amount and rate of weight loss are both considered. The second feature is dietary intake in relation to the patient's usual pattern. The patient is classified as having normal or abnormal intake; the duration and degree of abnormal intake is then noted. The third feature assessed is the presence of significant gastrointestinal symptoms such as anorexia, nausea, vomiting or diarrhea. 'Significant' indicates that these symptoms have persisted on a daily basis for two weeks or longer. The fourth feature considered is the patient's functional capacity or energy level. The last feature concerns the metabolic demands of any underlying disease state. This may range from a no-stress, physical situation to a high level of stress.

The physical exam then assesses loss of subcutaneous fat, muscle wasting, ankle edema, sacral edema and ascites. These are ranked as normal (0), mild (1+), moderate (2+), or severe (3+).

Once the history and physical exam are complete the dietitian can identify an SGA rank to indicate the patient's nutritional status (Detsky *et al.*, 1987). The categories include:

- well-nourished
- moderate or suspected malnutrition
- severe malnutrition.

It is important to note that in the assignment of a rank, one does not employ an explicit numerical weighting scheme, but rather a truly subjective weighting. The heaviest emphasis tends to be placed on weight loss, poor dietary intake, loss of subcutaneous tissue and muscle wasting.

# Assessment of pertinent lab values

Several lab values are useful in the overall assessment of nutritional status. Creatinine height index is an accurate measurement of somatic protein. Creatinine is a waste product of muscle metabolism and is excreted in the urine. The amount of creatinine produced is directly related to the amount of muscle present. As the amount of lean body mass decreases so does urinary creatinine excretion. By comparing actual urinary creatinine excreted over 24 hours to the expected excretion for height, deficits in lean body mass may be estimated. The expected values are 18 mg per kg of ideal body weight for females and 23 mg per kg ideal body weight for males. The creatinine height index is expressed as the actual-to-ideal ratio. Percentage deficit in creatinine/height index equals 100 minus actual urinary creatinine divided by ideal urinary creatinine, multiplied by 100.

$$\text{deficit in creatinine/height index} = 100 - \frac{\text{actual urinary creatinine}}{\text{ideal urinary creatinine}} \times 100$$

Blood work may be done to assess the visceral protein compartment. The three tests that may be used include serum albumin, serum transferrin and total lymphocyte count. Serum albumin as a parameter to assess serum protein status is directly quantified as part of the routine blood work. Normal levels of serum albumin range from 3.5–5 g/dl. Serum transferrin is a protein produced in the liver, that is assessed to determine visceral protein function. It is considered a more sensitive indicator of protein–calorie malnutrition than serum albumin (Miller Kovach, 1982). Normal levels of serum transferrin range from 2.31 to 4.32 g/l. Total lymphocyte count is used to measure immune function. Total lymphocyte counts of less than 2000/cu mm correlate well with the depressed immune function found in protein–calorie malnutrition.

Another blood test that is important, especially for individuals with bulimia nervosa is serum potassium. Normal potassium levels range from 3.5 to 5.5 meq/L. An individual who is routinely purging will have a lower-than-ideal potassium level, which could have potentially serious cardiac effects.

The actual lab tests done for different individuals will vary, depending on the severity of the weight loss. The physician involved in the case generally will have ordered the pertinent lab tests prior to referring the patient to a dietitian for nutritional assessment. If this has not been done it is important for the dietitian to communicate with the physician to request the appropriate lab tests.

# Calculation of treatment plan weights

For treatment purposes it is helpful to use specified weights to define the patient's state of nutritional well-being. In order for the patient to be a suitable candidate for outpatient treatment, it is essential that she be above what is considered a reasonable ambulatory weight. The designated weights are as follows: ideal weight, safe weight, activity or exercise weight, ambulatory weight and critical weight. These designated weights are presented in Box 2.2.

---

**Box 2.2:** *Designated weights for recovery program*

- *Ideal weight*: calculated using body mass index (BMI), and considering premorbid weight status for adults. Appropriate weight for height (NCHS percentiles for adolescents)
- *Safe weight*: calculated as 90% of ideal weight. Weight at which most persons may enjoy normal health status
- *Activity weight*: calculated as 80% of ideal weight. Appropriate for normal activities of daily living, not strenuous exercise
- *Ambulatory weight*: calculated as 75% of ideal weight. Very modest level of activity only
- *Critical weight*: calculated at 65% of ideal weight. Requires hospitalization and immediate medical and nutritional intervention

---

We must first consider ideal weight, as it is the basis from which all the others are derived. Ideal weight is calculated differently for adults than it is for adolescents. The ideal weight for an adult is calculated by use of BMI. BMI is arrived at by dividing the weight in kg by the height in meters squared. BMI of 20–25 is considered healthy. To come up with a more precise range, it is important to consider the individual's premorbid weight. This is because if the premorbid BMI was 24, for example, it will be very stressful for that individual to eventually try to maintain a BMI of 20 with normal healthy eating habits. An individual who has to restrict her intake in any way to maintain a certain weight will not be able to recover from her eating disorder. A case which demonstrates this point is as follows.

**Case study**
Anna was 28 years old when seen for assessment of her eating disorder. She was 170 cm tall, and her current weight was 50 kg. Prior to developing an eating disorder, her weight had been 68–69 kg for several years. This represented a BMI of 23.5–24, within the healthy range. At the time of assessment she pleaded with the therapist to set her ideal weight at 60 kg which represented a BMI of 20. When Anna started eating normally again, her weight fairly quickly went past 60 kg. She began to feel fat and like a failure, and once again started to restrict her intake. She was only able to be successful in normalizing her eating once a realistic ideal weight of 68 kg was accepted.

BMI is not a reliable way to set ideal weight for adolescents, due to their developmental stage. A more reliable method is by use of valid growth charts such as those developed by the NCHS. Ideal weight may be ascertained by plotting height on the growth chart appropriate for gender and age, and then choosing the weight that corresponds to the percentile that the height is on. As mentioned previously, it is important to consider previous linear growth patterns if growth stunting has occurred. An example of this would occur if the height of the patient being assessed was currently at the 10th percentile but this individual had been growing along the 25th percentile prior to developing an eating disorder. In this case the ideal weight would be deemed to be the weight for age on the 25th percentile, even though current height is at the 10th percentile. A situation which requires somewhat different consideration occurs when dealing with females between 16–18 years old who happen to be very tall. The corresponding weights on the NCHS growth charts tend to be unacceptably high. In this situation one should consider premorbid weight-gain patterns when setting ideal weight. To express actual weight as a percentage of ideal weight, divide actual weight by calculated ideal weight and multiply the answer by 100. A percentage of ideal weight of less than 75% is considered severely depleted, 75–85% is defined as depleted and over 85% is considered within the normal range.

In developing a nutritional treatment plan, a slightly more precise categorization of weights is used. Safe weight is calculated as 90% of ideal weight. Activity or exercise weight is 80% of ideal weight. For treatment purposes this includes normal activities of daily living, including moderate exercise, i.e. walking to school. It does not include strenuous activities such as competitive sports. Ambulatory weight, i.e. a weight which would usually allow outpatient treatment and not require hospitalization is 75% of ideal weight. Any individual with a weight below 75% of ideal would require hospitalization with medical intervention. Critical weight is a weight which would place the patient at serious risk both nutritionally and medically. Critical weight is calculated as 65% of ideal weight. Patients with body weights in this category require hospitalization and immediate medical and nutritional intervention, such as enteral or tube feeding. It must be kept in mind that these are values that are appropriate for the majority of patients; however, medical assessment always takes precedence. In other words, there may be individuals assessed to be at 80% of ideal weight whose medical status would demand hospitalization and possibly even bedrest. These calculated weights then are the general rule only. Individual medical assessment is crucial.

# Conclusion

Chapter 2 has presented the multidimensional model of eating disorders from four perspectives: the psychologist, the family therapist, the physician and the dietitian. These perspectives vary in terms of professional expertise, etiological focus and specific assessment tools. However, the underlying view vis à vis the patient-centered approach is the same; that clinicians must look at multiple factors (including sociocultural context, individual predispositions, family situation, trauma and biological/physiological factors) which play a role in developing and maintaining an eating disorder in the unique life of an individual.

# References

American Psychiatric Association (1994) *Diagnostic and Statistical Manual of Mental Disorders* (4e). APA, Washington DC.

American Psychiatric Association (2000) Practice guidelines for the treatment of patients with eating disorders (revision). *Am J Psychiatry.* **157** (Supplement): 1–39.

Andersen AE, Bowers W and Evans K (1997) Inpatient treatment of anorexia nervosa. In: DM Garner and PE Garfinkel (eds) *Handbook of Treatment for Eating Disorders* (2e). Guilford Press, New York.

Beck AT, Rush A, Shaw BF and Emery G (1979) *Cognitive Therapy of Depression.* Guilford Press, New York.

Bruch H (1973) *Eating Disorders: obesity, anorexia nervosa and the person within.* Basic Books, New York.

Bruch H (1978) *The Golden Cage.* Harvard University Press, Cambridge, MA.

Calam R, Waller G, Slade P and Newton T (1990) Eating disorders and perceived relationships with parents. *Int J Eat Disord.* **9**: 479–85.

Campbell TL (1986) Family's impact on health: a critical review. *Fam Syst Med.* **4**: 2–3.

Casper RC (1998) Behavioral activation and lack of concern, core symptoms of anorexia nervosa. *Int J Eat Disord.* **24**: 381–93.

Cassidy SB (1997) Prader-Willi syndrome. *J Med Genet.* **34**: 917–23.

Connors ME and Morse W (1993) Sexual abuse and eating disorders: a review. *Int J Eat Disord.* **13**: 1–11.

Dansky BS, Brewerton TD, Kilpatrick DG and O'Neil PM (1997) The National Women's Study: relationship of victimization and post-traumatic stress disorder to bulimia nervosa. *Int J Eat Disord.* **21**: 213–28.

Dare C and Eisler I (1997) Family therapy for anorexia nervosa. In: D Garner and P Garfinkel (eds) *Handbook of Treatment for Eating Disorders* (2e). Guilford Press, New York.

Dare C, Le Grange D, Eisler I and Rutherford J (1994) Redefining the psychosomatic family: family process of 26 eating-disordered families. *Int J Eat Disord.* **16**: 211–26.

Deep AL, Lilenfeld LR, Plotnicov KH, Pollice C and Kaye WH (1999) Sexual abuse in eating disorder subtypes and control women: the role of co-morbid substance dependence in bulimia nervosa. *Int J Eat Disord.* **25**: 1–10.

Detsky AS, McLaughlin JR, Baker JP *et al.* (1987) What is subjective global assessment of nutritional status? *J Parenter Enteral Nutr.* **11**(1): 8–13.

Fairburn CG and Cooper PJ (1984) The clinical feature of bulimia nervosa. *Br J Psychiatry.* **144**: 238–46.

Fairburn CG, Welch SL, Doll HA, Davies BA and O'Connor ME (1997) Risk factors for bulimia nervosa: a community-based case-control study. *Arch Gen Psychiatry.* **54**: 509–17.

Frisancho AE (1974) Triceps skinfold and upper arm muscle size norms for assessment of nutritional status. *Am J Clin Nutr.* **27**: 1052.

Garfinkel PE and Garner D (1982) *Anorexia Nervosa: a multidimensional perspective.* Brunner/Mazel, New York.

Garfinkel PE and Kaplan AS (1986) Anorexia nervosa: diagnostic conceptualizations. In: KD Brownell and JP Foreyt (eds) *Handbook of Eating Disorders.* Basic Books, New York.

Garner DM (1997) Psychoeducational principles in treatment. In: DM Garner and PE Garfinkel (eds) *Handbook of Treatment for Eating Disorders* (2e). Guilford Press, New York.

Garner DM and Bemis KM (1982) A cognitive-behavioral approach to anorexia nervosa. *Cogn Therapy Res.* **6**: 123–50.

Garner DM, Vitousek KM and Pike KM (1997) Cognitive-behavioral therapy for anorexia nervosa. In: DM Garner and PE Garfinkel (eds) *Handbook of Treatment for Eating Disorders*. Guilford Press, New York.

Gilligan C (1982) *In a Different Voice*. Harvard University Press, Cambridge, MA.

Gleaves DH, Eberenz KP and May MC (1998) Scope and significance of post-traumatic symptomatology among women hospitalized for an eating disorder. *Int J Eat Disord.* **24**: 147–56.

Goodsitt A (1985) Self-psychology and the treatment of anorexia nervosa. In: D Garner and PE Garfinkel (eds) *Handbook of Psychotherapy of Anorexia Nervosa and Bulimia*. Guilford Press, New York.

Gupta N, Ahmed K and Kulig J (1996) A sleepy, hungry teenager. *Adolesc Med.* **7**(3): 369–77.

Hahn NJ (1998) When food becomes a cry for help. *J Am Diet Assoc.* **98**(4): 395–8.

Haley J (1980) *Leaving Home: the therapy of disturbed young people*. McGraw-Hill, New York.

Hall L and Cohn L (1999) *Bulimia: a guide to recovery*. Gurze Books, Carlsbad, CA.

Hamill PVV, Drizd TA, Johnson CL *et al.* (1979) Physical growth: National Center for Health Statistics percentiles. *Am J Clin Nutr.* **32**: 607–29.

Hannun JW and Mayer JM (1984) Validation of two family assessment approaches. *J Marriage Fam.* **46**: 741–8.

Herzog DB and Copeland PM (1985) Eating disorders. *NEJM.* **313**(5): 295–303.

Hewitt PL, Flett GL and Ediger E (1995) Perfectionism traits and perfectionistic self-presentation in eating disorder attitudes, characteristics, and symptoms. *Int J Eat Disord.* **18**: 317–26.

Hoek HW (1997) Review of the epidemiological studies of eating disorders. *Int Rev Psychiatry.* **5**: 61–74.

Hornbacher M (1998) *Wasted*. Harper Collins, New York.

Humphrey LL (1991) Object relations and the family system: an integrative approach to understanding and treating eating disorders. In: CL Johnson (ed.) *Psychodynamic Treatment of Anorexia Nervosa and Bulimia*. Guilford Press, New York.

Jasper K (1993) Out from under the body image disparagement. In: C Brown and K Jasper (eds), *Consuming Passions: feminist approaches to weight preoccupation and eating disorders*. Second Story Press, Toronto, Canada.

Johnson CL (ed.) (1991) *Psychodynamic Treatment of Anorexia Nervosa and Bulimia*. Guilford Press, New York.

Kaplan AS (1993) Medical and nutritional assessment. In: AS Kaplan and PE Garfinkel (eds) *Medical Issues and the Eating Disorders: the interface*. Brunner/Mazel, New York.

Katzman MA and Waller G (1998) Implications of therapist gender in the treatment of eating disorders: daring to ask the questions. In: W Vandereycken (ed.) *The Burden of the Therapist*. Athelone Press, London, UK.

Kilbourne J (1994) Still killing us softly: advertising and the obsession with thinness. In: P Fallon, MA Katzman and SC Wooley (eds) *Feminist Perspectives on Eating Disorders*. Guilford Press, New York.

Kog E and Vandereycken W (1985) Family characteristics of anorexia and bulimia: a review of the research literature. *Clin Psychol Rev.* **5**: 159–80.

Kog E and Vandereycken W (1989) Family interaction in eating disorder patients and normal controls. *Inter J Eat Disord.* **8**: 11–23.

Krug-Wispe S (1993) Nutritional assessment. In: PM Queen and CE Long (eds) *Handbook of Pediatric Nutrition*. Aspen Publishers Inc, Gaithersburg, MD.

Le Grange D (1999) Family therapy for adolescent anorexia nervosa. *J Clin Psychology.* **55**: 727–39.

Le Grange D, Eisler I, Dare C and Hodes M (1992) Family criticism and self-starvation: a study of expressed emotion. *J Fam Therapy.* **14**: 177–92.

Levine P (1996) Eating disorders and their impact on family systems. In: F Kaslow (ed.) *Handbook of Relational Diagnosis and Dysfunctional Family Patterns*. John Wiley & Sons, New York.

Mather SA (1997) *Leaving Food Behind*. Mather Publications For Growth and Wellness, Inc, Nepean, ON.

Miller D (1994) *Women Who Hurt Themselves: a book of hope and understanding*. Basic Books, New York.

Miller Kovach K (1982) The assessment of nutritional status in anorexia nervosa. In: Meir Gross (ed.) *Anorexia Nervosa*. The Collamore Press, Toronto, ON, Canada.

Minuchin S, Rosman BL and Baker L (1978) *Psychosomatic Families: anorexia nervosa in context*. Harvard University Press, Cambridge, MA.

Morgan JF, Reid F and Lacey JH (1999) The SCOFF questionnaire: assessment of a new tool for eating disorders. *BMJ.* **319**: 1467–8.

Pipher M (1994) *Reviving Ophelia: saving the selves of adolescent girls*. Random House, Toronto, ON, Canada.

Mills D (1989) Recommended nutrient intakes for Canadians. In: *Ontario Dietetic Association, Ontario Hospital Association Nutritional Care Manual*. Ontario Hospital Association, Ontario, Canada.

Reiff DW and Lampson Reiff KK (1992) *Eating Disorders Nutrition Therapy in the Recovery Process*. Aspen Publishers Inc, Gathersburg, MD.

Robin AL, Siegel PT, Koepke T, Moye AW and Tice S (1994) Family therapy versus individual therapy for adolescent females with anorexia nervosa. *J Dev Behav Pediatr.* **15**: 111–6.

Root M, Fallon P and Fredrich W (1986) *Bulimia: a systems approach to treatment*. Norton, New York.

Schwartz RC and Barrett MJ (1988) Woman and eating disorders. *J Psychother Fam.* 6: 89–105.

Schwartz RC and Grace P (1990) The systemic treatment of bulimia. *J Psychother Fam.* 6: 89–105.

Selvini-Palazzoli M and Viaro M (1988) The anorectic process in the family: a six-stage model as a guide for individual therapy. *Fam Process.* 27: 129–48.

Shugar G and Kruger S (1995) Aggressive family communication, weight gain and improved eating attitudes during systemic family therapy for anorexia nervosa. *Int J Eat Disord.* 17: 23–31.

Sours JA (1980) *Starving to Death in a Sea of Objects.* Jason Aranson, New York.

Steiner-Adair C (1994) The politics of prevention. In: PA Fallon, MA Katzman and SC Wooley (eds) *Feminist Perspectives on Eating Disorders.* Guilford Press, New York.

Strober M (1997) Consultation and therapeutic engagement in severe anorexia nervosa. In: DM Garner and PE Garfinkel (eds) *Handbook of Treatment for Eating Disorders.* Guilford Press, New York.

Strober M and Humphrey LL (1987) Familial contributions to the etiology and course of anorexia nervosa and bulimia. *J Consult Clin Psychol.* 55: 654–9.

Strober M, Lampert C, Morrell W, Burroughs J and Jacobs C (1990) A controlled family study of anorexia nervosa: evidence of familial aggregation and lack of shared transmission with affective disorders. *Int J Eat Disord.* 9: 239–53.

Thompson C (1996) The voices from within. Available at www.mirror-mirror.org (website for eating disorders).

Thompson DA, Berg KM and Shatford LA (1987) The heterogeneity of bulimic symptomatology: cognitive and behavioral dimensions. *Int J Eat Disord.* 6: 215–34.

Thompson JK, Coovert MD, Richards KJ, Johnson, S and Cattarin J (1995) Development of body image, eating disturbance, and general psychological functioning in female adolescents: covariance structure modeling and longitudinal investigations. *Int J Eat Disord.* 18: 221–36.

Waller G and Katzman MA (1997) Female or male therapists for women with eating disorders?: a pilot study of expert opinions. *Int J Eat Disord.* 22: 111–14.

White M (1983) Anorexia nervosa: a transgenerational system perspective. *Fam Process.* 22(3): 255–73.

White M (1987) Anorexia nervosa: a cybernetic perspective. *Fam Therapy Collect.* 20: 117–29.

Wiseman CV, Gray JJ, Mosimann JE and Ahrens AH (1992) Cultural expectation of thinness in women: an update. *Int J Eat Disord.* 11: 85–9.

Wiseman CV, Harris WA and Halmi KA (1998) Eating disorders. *Med Clin North Am.* 82: 145–59.

Wolf N (1991) *The Beauty Myth.* Vintage Books, Toronto, Canada.

Zerbe KJ (1993) *The Body Betrayed: women, eating disorders and treatment.* American Psychiatric Press, Washington DC.

# 3

# The illness experience: eating disorders from the patient's perspective

*Kathleen M Berg*

Central to any comprehensive understanding of eating disorders are the subjective experiences of those who have suffered through anorexia nervosa and bulimia nervosa. It is surprising, therefore, that researchers and clinicians have paid comparatively little attention to the patient's voice in their attempts to understand the development of and process of recovery from these complex, often recalcitrant disorders (Hsu *et al.*, 1992; Rorty *et al.* 1993; Serpell *et al.*, 1999). Some authors (Vitousek *et al.*, 1991) have noted how difficult it is to obtain accurate self-reports in disorders where the patient's internal experience may be misrepresented through denial, distortion and a lack of interoceptive awareness (difficulty identifying emotional and physiological states). This is particularly the case with patients suffering from anorexia nervosa. Despite these caveats, it is essential that clinicians and significant others seek to understand the subjective world of patients who suffer from eating disorders by focusing on autobiographical accounts of recovery, by interviewing those in recovery and by familiarizing themselves with the few qualitative studies available. This chapter explores the illness experience as revealed to us by the sufferers themselves. In particular, it examines the emotional experiences, ideas and opinions, impact on life experience and expectations of the clinician from the patient's perspective. In doing so, we seek to deepen our appreciation of their profound despair and expand our understanding of the factors they felt contributed to the development of their disorder, were central to the recovery process (both promoting and sabotaging) and increased their vulnerability to relapse.

# Emotional experience

When the primacy of the patient is recognized in healthcare, a more collaborative approach to treatment is encouraged. This approach acknowledges the wide variability in etiology, symptoms and symptom function, maintaining factors and treatment response for both anorexia nervosa and bulimia nervosa. Many patients decry the use of pejorative labels which fail to acknowledge their individuality and uniqueness of experience. Mather (1997) explained her reticence to seek help from the professional community: 'I always cringe when I hear a doctor or someone else describe a human being as a "bulimic". To me, that label is so shaming ... I couldn't stand to listen to someone define me by a clause or paragraph in a textbook.' Similarly, in her memoir entitled *Wasted*, Hornbacher (1998) asserts: 'I wrote this because I object to the homogenizing, the inaccurate trend in the majority of eating disorders literature that tends to generalize from the part to the whole, from a person to a group.' These reactions underscore the importance of looking beyond theoretical generalities, paying careful attention to the intimate details of each individual's emotional experience. Such an approach will foster the development of common ground and promote a stronger therapeutic alliance.

Exploration of a variety of feeling states helps to describe the emotional world of those who are struggling with anorexia nervosa and bulimia nervosa. A number of these feeling states are explored here, including: initial denials of pain and suffering and accompanying feelings of euphoria, shame and feelings of inferiority, fear and distrust, depression and longing, anger and grief.

# Euphoria and denial

Initial denials of suffering, particularly in anorexia nervosa, are often accompanied by a calm exterior, a smiling face and dismissals of any concerns regarding fatigue, emotional distress or hunger. It is interesting to note that many patients in recovery will later admit to deliberate deception. Common misconceptions expressed by clinicians and family/friends alike are the notions that the patient is demonstrating complacency with the disorder or that she is defending her self-starvation or binge/purge behavior as a deliberate attack on them. Some patients actually express considerable relief in response to a well-timed confrontation by a caring, knowledgeable clinician. Others defend their relentless pursuit of thinness vigorously and describe a sense of omnipotence with feelings of euphoria. In *The Art of Starvation*, for example, Sheila MacLeod states: 'Having disposed alike of unwanted flesh and unwanted menstruation, I had become pure and clean and therefore superior to those around me. I was so superior that I considered myself to be virtually beyond criticism' (MacLeod, 1981). The author goes on to note that although her inner euphoric state and demonstrations of supreme willpower created an illusion of being in control, she was amazed at how indiscernible her underlying terror of losing control was to parents, teachers and peers.

Many patients who have suffered from anorexia nervosa are able to articulate their own strategies for maintaining this euphoric state. For example, some patients convince themselves that the potential medical consequences of self-starvation apply to others but not to themselves. While patients may pay careful attention to this information and even express fear in the therapy session, some describe a process of mentally dismissing the information on their way out of the office. Subsequent to the session, they simply 'do not think about it'. In response to any intrusive thoughts which do not support food refusal, patients will often convince themselves that they will feel better if they don't eat. Indeed, many patients publicly state that weight loss is far more important to them than health. When questioned about fears of eventual death, patients may claim that they 'just don't believe it' or that 'It's only the really thin ones who die'. These cognitive strategies serve to maintain the euphoric state, especially in the initial phases of the disorder.

Those suffering from bulimia nervosa frequently explain their initial denials by referring to their own deep-seated shame and fear of rejection or to concerns about inflicting pain on loved ones. One patient put it this way:

'My mother has suffered enough in her life and I was trying to protect her from more pain. I didn't want to let her down. Besides, pigging out and barfing are just so disgusting. I just got really good at hiding it.'

# Shame and feelings of inferiority

Interview dialogues and autobiographical accounts reveal an underlying despair among those with eating disorders which is profound and deeply rooted. Shame and intense self-hatred are common themes with patients who engage in bingeing and purging behaviors. Many describe themselves as inherently defective, inferior and undeserving of the good things in life. Hornbacher (1998) hated her body with such 'incredible force that love of food was forced underground, my masochistic side surfaced and anorexia became my goal'.

Binge eating is described by these patients as disgusting, animalistic and out of control. During an art experience exercise conducted as part of group therapy for bulimia nervosa, one patient drew herself as a pig with the inscription, 'Here sits a worthless fat pig' scribbled below. This was the patient's response, in spite of instructions not to use stick figures or draw herself in symbolic form. In a recent study by Brooks *et al.* (1998), 10 women and one man were interviewed about their experiences with bulimia nervosa. All of the respondents marginalized their disorder and themselves. Bulimia nervosa was described as 'abnormal', 'revolting' and 'shameful'. Participants also marginalized themselves with derogatory terms including 'alien', 'freak' and 'disgusting creature'. In addition, they felt that they were the 'poor cousin' whereas anorexia nervosa (restricting type) was viewed as 'the ultimate'. In fact, one participant, Carmen, reported feeling 'more revolting' when placed in a support group with emaciated patients struggling with anorexia nervosa.

Purging behaviors are responded to with similar feelings of shame and embarrassment particularly for those who engage in self-induced vomiting. When confronted with evidence of self-induced vomiting, individuals will often say they have the flu or that they have food allergies. They may express surprise or confusion over their stomach's 'reaction to the food' or they may deny the vomiting altogether. Patients frequently comment that underlying these deceptions are feelings of tremendous guilt for being a 'fake' and a 'cheat' and deep shame for losing control.

At an even deeper level, most patients with eating disorders experience themselves as shameful for having even engaged in the act of eating. They feel unworthy for having needs and disgraced for trying to fulfill them. This may include needs for nourishment, attention, affection, sexual gratification or comfort. Many of the individuals who participated in the Brooks *et al.* (1998) interviews described bulimia nervosa as a personality defect. According to the respondents, this 'defectiveness' is demonstrated through low levels of willpower, self-discipline or self-control as evidenced by failures to stay on a diet.

The following case study of Ann demonstrates how one young woman incorporated perceived messages of inferiority and unworthiness into a self-concept infused with shame.

### Case study

Ann, aged 26, was a first-year medical resident who sought treatment for depression. During the initial assessment, Ann was questioned on any changes in her appetite and her current eating habits. She explained that she was a vegetarian, had a high metabolic rate and exercised regularly. She said that she often 'forgot' to eat because she was so busy but denied dieting or any problems with overeating. After several sessions, Ann revealed that she engaged in binge-eating episodes followed by self-induced vomiting or periods of highly restricted eating. She said that she had been afraid of rejection and too ashamed to discuss this earlier in therapy. Ann had a very negative self-concept. Despite her academic achievements, she did not view herself as intelligent and attributed her successes to luck or chance.

Ann was raised on a farm on the east coast of Canada. She described her mother as a sad, self-effacing woman devoted to her family, and her father as a hard-working, rather stoical man. She was the oldest of three children, having a younger brother, aged 22 and a sister aged 15 who was born with Down's syndrome. Ann described her early childhood as very happy. As she got older, however, she became acutely aware of her family's poverty and the financial and emotional strain which her parents experienced. Over time, Ann recalled feeling increasingly ashamed of wanting or needing anything. Her parents often became irritated if she requested their attention. Her father tended to chide her for emotional displays and her mother made frequent references to how lucky she was that she was born healthy, unlike her sister. Ann picked up the message that a good person is rational and self-sufficient and that emotionality is weak and selfish. Even though she learned to keep her feelings to herself, she knew that on the inside, she was deeply hurt and angry. She expressed shame both for her feelings and for her secret strong needs for attention and affection. To complicate matters, Ann spent four months as a volunteer in a Third World country during her undergraduate studies. Her response to this experience was to feel a heightened sense of shame for having what she called 'privileges I have not earned'. This came to include all things she deemed pleasurable or wasteful, including relaxation, new clothing, time for 'fun' and eventually food. She described feeling ashamed of her wants and her needs and of her body for having them. Food indulgences (these were often normal meals) resulted in self-induced vomiting, guilt and prayers that she would become a better person.

# Fear and distrust

Individuals with anorexia nervosa or bulimia nervosa are tormented by a pervasive fear of life and distrust of others. In describing her emotional recovery, Mather (1997) wrote:

'I was scared of life and everything in it. Although I didn't realize it at the time, fear was so much a part of my life that its absence would have created even more fear.'

Similarly, Hornbacher (1998) described herself as an apprehensive, vigilant child who felt the constant presence of something dark and threatening. She described her self-imposed isolation as an attempt to seek refuge from a world she perceived as fascinating but dangerous. While there is tremendous variation in the ways patients describe their fears, they can be organized under general themes which serve to facilitate the reader's appreciation of their breadth and depth of intensity. The themes explored here are:

- fear of fat
- fear of going out of control
- fear of change
- fear of emotional flooding
- fear of abandonment and loss of approval
- fear of clinical interventions and distrust of practitioners
- fear of losing the eating disorder as a coping strategy.

A study conducted by Rorty *et al.* (1993) used semi-structured interviews to investigate patients' beliefs regarding factors related to their recovery. The participants were 40 women who had recovered from bulimia nervosa for one year or more. Their findings indicated that the fear of getting fat and concomitant body-image disparagement/distortion were rated as the most difficult features of the eating disorder to change. Fears of weight gain are particularly debilitating to patients who were overweight as children and who suffered the rejection and humiliation inflicted on them by a weight-prejudiced society obsessed with thinness and perfection. One patient in treatment for anorexia nervosa gave an emotional account of being taunted and threatened by groups of children on her way to and from public school. She was called 'blubber-puss' and was frequently poked, pushed and chased. A standard joke among her harassers was that in the event of a famine, she could live off her own fat for decades. Another patient who had struggled for two years with bulimia nervosa described a similar experience in which boys would rate the bodies of girls lining up for lunch in the cafeteria on a scale of one to 10 and declare her a 'big fat zero'. This young woman became adamant that she would never go through that again.

Fear of going out of control is a related source of terror for patients with eating disorders. For Mather (1997), loss of control was terrifying in that being in control meant surviving. Most patients have rigid self-imposed rules about eating and fear going out of control around food. Many describe strategies they devised in order to control their appetites and hence their eating behavior. These strategies include chewing gum, smoking, drinking diet Coke and black coffee, drinking copious amount of water and constantly repeating statements to themselves like 'I am not hungry. I just have an upset stomach' or 'It's not time to eat yet. You'll feel better if you don't'. Patients claim that these strategies have a calming effect because they foster a feeling of being in control and hence boost self-esteem. Other patients develop intense fears of the food itself.

**Case study**
Courtney, aged 13, described having an anxiety reaction to any foods she believed were high in fat: 'Whenever I even think of eating fries or burgers

or pizza or anything with a lot of fat, I panic. I feel like the fat is going to suffocate me or make me vomit. Whenever people serve those foods at parties, I just have to get out of there. I'm terrified I'll pass out or throw up.'

For some patients, fears of any change in their routine are closely aligned with fears of loss of control. Patients have reported a variety of changes in their lives which elicit intense anxiety, contributing to onset of the disorder, exacerbation of existing symptoms or relapse. These include moving to a new city or neighborhood, changing schools, losing a good friend, separation/divorce of parents, entering high school or post-secondary education, moving away from home, starting a new job and beginning a romantic relationship. In addition, minor changes in routine which interfere with rituals to control food intake, exercise or purging may result in a strong anxiety reaction outwardly displayed as irritability. Examples given by patients include being interrupted by a visitor, being asked to run an errand, being required to eat with others, having a meal served at a different time and unavailability of the kinds of food they allow themselves to eat.

For many patients, an eating disorder provides refuge from intense feelings which they try to starve out, drown or swallow whole. Mather (1997) refers to these feelings as her warehouse of emotions. Over time, the container becomes too small to house the myriad of emotions and patients will often express fears of emotional flooding. In her memoirs, Hornbacher (1998) makes frequent references to her terror of her own needs and passions. It becomes increasingly difficult for the patient to tolerate the mounting intensity of her emotions. She will often express fears of being annihilated by them. In the author's experience, those with a history of trauma such as childhood sexual abuse are particularly fearful of affective flooding.

Fears of abandonment and loss of approval are exceptionally strong emotions for those suffering with anorexia nervosa and bulimia nervosa. According to Mather (1997), her fear of abandonment was at the heart of all her other fears. She felt that if abandoned, she would be alone, helpless and unable to survive. Patients have recounted many stories of how they developed an ability to 'psych out' a social gathering, searching for behavioral and verbal cues of 'acceptable' conduct. They would then mimic the gestures and verbal expressions in order to gain approval and fit in. When these patients are questioned about loss of personal authenticity and emotional distancing in their social interactions, they often state that loss of approval and others' perceptions are far more important than their own feelings. Furthermore, patients are often convinced that interpersonal closeness will result in abandonment: 'If I let him get to know the real me, I'll be rejected'. Hornbacher (1998) describes this fear in a powerful way: 'I was an anorectic because I was afraid of being human. Implicit in human contact is the exposure of the self, the interaction of selves.'

Fears of clinical interventions and distrust of practitioners are often expressed by those with eating disorders. On the Something Fishy Website on Eating Disorders (www.something-fishy.org), one author (Medina, 1998) compiled a list of fears patients expressed by e-mail in anticipation of reaching out for professional help. Unfortunately, much of the anxiety expressed is based on negative experiences with physicians and therapists wherein the patient's concerns were trivialized, minimized or dismissed altogether. Many patients expressed fears of not being believed or not taken seriously either because they were 'not thin enough', not physically sick enough, not the right age (frequently noted by those whose age exceeds 25) or not the right sex (a common fear expressed by males). Those affected by anorexia nervosa are frequently told 'Well, just eat' and those with bulimia nervosa are advised to 'Just stop when you're full'. In the authors' experience, sufferers and their parents/partners have been exasperated by comments like: 'This is just a phase all teenage girls go through. She'll grow out of it'. On more than one occasion, patients have written to the author in advance of their initial consultation, begging to be taken seriously.

At the other end of the spectrum are those who fear being diagnosed as 'crazy'. Fodor (1997) expressed this fear as follows: 'I refused to seek professional counseling because I was certain that either I would be committed to a mental institution or put on display as a freak of nature for scientists around the world to study.'

Another commonly expressed fear is that the doctor or therapist is going to make the patient get fat or gain weight. Recently, reports are surfacing from women who were hospitalized with eating disorders in the 1980s. A number of them describe situations in which they were forced to eat, felt hated by the nursing staff and ignored by the therapists. One woman recently told the author that she kept her weight up to avoid enduring the hospital experience again. The failure to acknowledge and legitimize the patient's feelings leads to a no-win situation for both the sufferer and the caregiver. This predicament is well-documented by Monika Ostroff (Hall and Ostroff, 1999) in her account of sessions with a hospital therapist:

'I tried to talk about my anxiety which stemmed from the tube calories and how scared I was to eat, but he wouldn't let me, telling me that discussions about food and weight were off limits. Suddenly I felt ashamed that I had these fears. He went on to tell me that all anorexics are manipulative. Listening to him made me feel backed into a corner. What could I do with my anxiety if I couldn't talk about it? I managed it by continuing not to eat from the trays.'

Closely related to fears of clinical intervention are the patient's concerns about losing her eating disorder as a coping strategy. When a disorder is viewed as a guardian (Serpell et al., 1999), it takes on the status of protector and source of security, the 'thing you believe is keeping you safe, alive, contained ...' (Hornbacher, 1998). Knowledge of this dynamic greatly enhances one's appreciation of the intense fears patients encounter when confronting treatments which require them to relinquish their starvation or binge/purge behaviors.

# Depression and spiritual longing

The euphoria experienced in the initial phases of an eating disorder eventually gives way to depression. In describing her own journey through anorexia nervosa, MacLeod (1981) states that her own depression did not actually follow euphoria but was masked by it; that early experiences of self-confidence combined with high energy levels eventually collapsed and despair emerged. MacLeod explains that bearing and denying her depression at the same time was an attempt to cope publicly with the shame of defeat (defined by weight gain, going off a diet, etc.) which she found unbearable. She began to seek comfort in depression itself with the same willpower and determination evidenced by her self-starvation.

Many patients with anorexia nervosa are very high on endurance and express pride in their ability to suffer emotional and physical pain. Despite this, there is a self underneath who is desperate to be rescued from the torment.

Patients who have been affected by bulimia nervosa also speak of 'hitting rock bottom' (Rorty et al., 1993). Fodor (1997) speaks of reaching an all-time low and feeling emotionally burned-out. By the age of 25, Mather (1997) felt as though she was just existing and trying to get through each day, having lost contact with her desire to learn, her zest for life and her sense of humor.

Eating disorders have been described by some as a passive form of suicide. In the acute phases of the disorder, some patients, especially those who have experienced innumerable hospitalizations and outpatient treatments, contemplate suicide in response to feelings of hopelessness. However, the expressed intent to commit suicide is, in the author's experience, rare. MacLeod (1981) notes that although she wrote in her diary that she wished she were dead, she never seriously considered suicide as a solution to her problems. As one who has recovered from anorexia nervosa, she does not consider self-starvation and attempted suicide as synonymous. Similarly, Hornbacher (1998) asserts that clinicians are overfocused on the end result of self-starvation and binge/purge cycles when the patient is depressed, passive and helpless. She claims that her initial intention was to rise above all adversity to become strong and survive the oppressive forces in her life. Having said this, it is vitally important to reiterate that the lives of those suffering from eating disorders are varied and complex. For example, many patients are also struggling with a history of childhood sexual abuse, alcohol/drug addictions or emotional/physical abuse.

These experiences can be the initial basis for or exacerbate existing depression and create a heightened risk for suicide.

In addition to depression, some patients also report strong spiritual longings and a search for deeper meaning in their lives. Patients have described this longing in various ways including 'a deep and insatiable hunger in our collective unconscious' (Hornbacher, 1998), an attempt to 'connect with the spiritual world through food' (Mather, 1997) and as one patient recently put it 'a search for the inner meaning of my life that is separate from what everyone else wants me to do.' According to Normandi and Roark (1998), both of whom have survived eating disorders, spiritual wounds co-exist with physical and emotional wounds in the development and maintenance of obsessions with food and weight. Roark states that 'Thinness was my god and I was on a spiritual quest' (Normandi and Roark, 1998). The writers claim that their eating disorders represented that part of their soul crying out for a deeper connection with the spiritual self in a culture that worships money, power, success and thinness. The author has also spoken to several patients who have described their dieting and fasting as attempts to achieve spiritual purity and worthiness. Some have used food refusal as a way to atone for their 'sins'. They feel that 'overeating' is a failure to resist temptation and is unclean. Rigid dietary codes, self-denial and ritualistic behavior around food become ways to make up for their 'transgressions'.

# Anger and grief

In general, the anger experienced by patients with eating disorders can be divided into three categories: anger toward self, anger toward the disorder and anger toward others. Anger toward self is described, in part, in the section on shame and feelings of inferiority. Patients express anger toward themselves for a myriad of 'transgressions', including:

- failure to stay on a diet
- having a body size or shape that does not conform to the cultural ideal of beauty
- being larger than peers or siblings
- perceived weakness in needing love or nourishment
- possessing a survival instinct that defends a biologically normal body weight
- imperfections in performance (academic, athletic or social) and letting others down.

A great deal of this self-directed anger is inflicted on the body as exemplified in the following case study.

**Case study**
Simone, aged 14, was referred for individual psychotherapy when her mother discovered bags of vomit under her bed. At the age of 12, she had been diagnosed with anorexia and spent four weeks in the hospital. She was discharged when her weight reached 100 lbs, a number she continued to view as magical in terms of the 'safety' it provided. To Simone, weighing 100 lbs meant that her weight was not low enough to be re-hospitalized; nor was she in danger of becoming 'fat'. On discharge, Simone continued with the food plan prescribed by her dietitian and her weight increased to 105 lbs. She reported feeling shocked as she expected her weight to stabilize at 100 lbs if she stuck to the food plan. She was angry at the hospital staff and felt she had been deceived. Her response was to cut down on portions and skip lunch. Unable to cope with these restrictions, she began to binge-eat when the family was not at home. She discovered self-induced vomiting as a way to keep her weight down. Simone became very astute at hiding the evidence of her bingeing and purging and this behavior continued for about six months. She reported feeling very angry at herself for 'going out of control', for having a 'dark secret' and for 'hurting' her parents. Simone felt compelled to punish herself by punching her thighs whenever she engaged in binge/purge episodes. On several occasions she had used a razor to make three cuts on her left hip. Simone explained that these wounds were a reminder of how 'bad' she had been and a message to 'smarten up'. She despised her body for needing food and was angry at its reaction to receiving it (bloating, weight gain, constipation). She wanted to feel empty, claiming that this was the only thing that comforted her. Simone's body had become the battleground for all her inner torment and self-hatred.

Hornbacher (1998) describes the vehemence with which hatred of one's body is experienced by those struggling with an eating disorder: 'You cross over from a vague wish to be thinner into a no-holds-barred attack on your flesh.'

Some patients reify the eating disorder itself and harbor intense hatred toward it. There is a tendency to demonize the disorder and to view it as a powerful monster which has taken over and ruined their lives (Brooks *et al.*, 1998; Serpell *et al.*, 1999). The patient begins to feel victimized and betrayed by a disorder which in the beginning was perceived as a benevolent safety net.

At the beginning of recovery, other-directed anger is disavowed in many sufferers. Anger toward others and grief over the loss of the eating disorder tend to be emergent issues over the course of recovery. In the earlier phases of treatment most patients are more likely to promote personal blame and protect parents, siblings, partners, etc. Initially, other-directed anger is more likely to be explicitly expressed towards professionals. This is particularly true of anorexia nervosa patients who have been brought in for treatment and are not self-referred. The professional is perceived to be the enemy who is weighing, feeding and placing restrictions on her. Practitioners may be viewed as interfering sabo-teurs who are trying to make the patient fat, robbing her of autonomy.

As the behaviors which served to numb out emotional responses are relin-quished, buried feelings often rise to the surface. Patients begin to recognize and express previously denied or suppressed emotions. Rage over physical and sexual abuse or betrayals by friends may emerge. Anger toward parents for fail-ing to acknowledge the patient's right to her authentic self and toward society for cultural pressures regarding thinness and perfection are increasingly expressed. In discussing the emergence of her own 'internalized' rage, Mather (1997) explains that she 'swallowed' her anger because she feared the possible abandon-ment and rejection resulting from its expression. Moreover, accessing her emo-tions created ambivalence over what emerged; rage and contempt toward her parents. Mather later recognized that in curtailing her anger through bingeing and starving, she allowed it to fester and grow. She also describes the ways in which she learned to displace her disowned rage and resentment; by breaking things, by manipulating others or denigrating them, by refusing to do favors and by resisting any attempts to help her.

In re-accessing their emotional lives, patients begin to experience a powerful grieving process. They become increasingly aware of the losses they have suf-fered as a result of their eating disorder. Patients begin to talk about diminished physical health and vitality (including possible fertility problems), loss of friends and lovers, interference with educational/career prospects and damage to family relationships (Serpell *et al.*, 1999). This is an extremely painful time for patients who have already suffered immensely and worked extremely hard to 'achieve' the very situation they now struggle to emancipate themselves from. However, in spite of the long and arduous journey, many of those who have recovered offer encouraging words about the reclaiming to their emotional selves. Lindsay Hall (Hall and Cohn, 1999) shares her own feelings on this: 'As weird as it may sound, my bulimia is responsible for who and where I am today, because without such a serious illness, I might never have worked so hard to be happy. I had to overcome every barrier that was in my way so that I could live and love fully, with my own set of values and ideals.'

# Ideas and opinions

## Myths and misconceptions about eating disorders: patient views

Patients have very definite views on myths and misconceptions about the etiol-ogy, treatment and recovery of anorexia nervosa and bulimia nervosa. These beliefs tend to be uniquely individual and sometimes disparate.

**Myth 1:** 'Eating disorders are just a stage of development girls go through. They will grow out of it'

Despite the increased media attention on eating disorders, patients and their families continue to be exasperated by family physicians and counselors who view excessive exercising, dieting and binge-eating as part of a 'normal' phase of adolescent development. Indeed, Hornbacher (1998) claims that this misconception of eating-disordered behavior as a passing phase was a major impetus for writing her memoirs. Rose (personal communication, 1999) also points out the dangers inherent in this kind of minimization. The misunderstanding that the disorder is a conscious choice, that it is nothing but 'vanity in action' and that one can simply choose to re-exercise control over it at will serves to alienate the patient and add to her feelings of hopelessness. Conversely, others (i.e. Hornbacher, 1998) are adverse to theories which tell the patient that she is powerless over her disorder. Hornbacher's belief is that this message is dangerous because it exonerates the patient of responsibility: 'I liked sitting back in my chair, chain-smoking, sighing with relief and thinking this is beyond my control' (Hornbacher, 1998).

Contrary to simplistic notions about eating disorders, most patients believe that they are multicausal in nature. Rose (personal communication, 1999) speaks of perfectionism, strong needs for approval, low self-esteem, social pressures to be thin and dysfunctional family patterns in discussing the etiology of her battle with anorexia nervosa. Hornbacher (1998) refers to high parental expectations, a perfectionistic personality, emotional blunting by adults and the search for a personality as factors contributing to the development of her eating disorder.

**Myth 2:** 'Anorexia nervosa is an attempt to avoid growing up'

Patients express varying opinions regarding the theory that anorexia nervosa represents a fear of the maturational process and a desire to return to a pre-adolescent state. Most objections refer to the idea that these patients are trying to avoid the mature responsibilities of adult life. On the contrary, patients report that they have shouldered adult responsibilities like caregiver, nurturer and peacemaker from a very young age.

For some patients ambivalence about growing up is related to the development of their bodies. For example, Rose (personal communication, 1999) felt unprepared for the sudden sexual development of her body, particularly the expansion of her hips and breasts. She wanted to retrieve the thin 'sexless' body which her parents and ballet teachers had approved of. Moreover, maintaining a thin body was a protection against being viewed as a sexual being. Other patients have commented on their belief that being tiny, cute and child-like in appearance made them special particularly in the eyes of their fathers;

they became reluctant to give up this perceived status. MacLeod (1981) believes that her self-starvation was an avoidance of the roles attached to womanhood; roles she learned represented passivity, a loss of self and sexual objectification. She saw the cessation of her menstrual cycle as a major achievement and viewed girlhood as a much safer existence. In contrast, Hornbacher's (1998) belief is that anorexia nervosa is an attempt to emancipate oneself from the nest; a mission not to need love and comfort. Furthermore, she rejects the view that self-starvation is always a desperate attempt to stave off signs of sexual maturity. Hornbacher states that she was not afraid of sex but ashamed that it fascinated her. Both Hornbacher and MacLeod believe that fears of budding sexuality may be more related to the culture's ambiguous and conflicted view of female sexuality.

**Myth 3:** 'Anorexia nervosa and bulimia nervosa are essentially about food and weight issues'

According to those who have struggled through eating disorders, the propagation of this myth has resulted in treatment approaches focussed largely on weight gain and external control of bingeing and purging behavior to the relative exclusion of attending to emotional and spiritual wounds. In *It's Not About Food*, the authors discuss their belief that ending obsessions with food and weight requires an approach which goes beyond the physical act of eating: 'It is a process of reaching deep into your own insatiable emotional and spiritual hunger, that which you have been trying to satisfy with food' (Normandi and Roark, 1998). Rose (personal communication, 1999) points to a number of misunderstandings related to her treatment needs in recovery. These included: the notion that the dissemination of information regarding medical consequences would curb self-starvation, the failure to understand the personal (emotional) 'hell' she was going through and failure to comprehend the 'eating disorder voice' which drives and torments the sufferer. Clearly, many patients are telling us that treatment approaches which focus solely on food and weight issues are inadequate.

**Myth 4:** 'Individuals with eating disorders don't feel'

Girls and women with eating disorders become adept at denying emotional and physical pain. Self- or other-imposed rules for social conduct include a smiling face, a pleasant disposition and behavior which conforms to social norms and accommodates the needs of others. Confronted with this outward appearance, clinicians and family members alike may develop two common misconceptions; that the individual is just fine and their concerns are exaggerated or that the individual is cold and unfeeling. The latter belief is heightened when they observe the periods of irritability and social isolation common to eating disorders. Patients in recovery are quick to challenge this myth. Hall (Hall and Cohn, 1999) speaks of her underlying tension, guilt, desperation and loneliness. Mather (1997) states that her cycles of bingeing, purging and starving served to keep intense feelings down and that the process exhausted her. According to Rose (personal communication, 1999), her anorexia nervosa and self-injurious behavior served to numb her emotional pain and keep her anger toward others buried. The stress of keeping these feelings silent becomes overwhelming as the eating disorder intensifies.

**Myth 5:** 'There are no cures for eating disorders. You just have to learn to live with them'

In Hornbacher's (1998) view, the classification of eating disorders as medical diseases is an unhelpful misconception. Patients and their families enter the therapeutic process looking for a 'cure' in the traditional sense. This belief is perpetuated by approaches which rely solely on medication and/or normalization of eating patterns. Hornbacher believes that the patient heals herself in collaboration with medication, therapy and support from family and friends. Several memoirs and guides to recovery have been written by individuals who have recovered from both anorexia nervosa (Hall and Ostroff, 1999; Hornbacher, 1998; MacLeod, 1981) and bulimia nervosa (Fodor, 1997; Hall and Cohn, 1999; Mather, 1997). Virtually all of these authors note that recovery is long-term and punctuated with relapses but it is definitely possible. When asked to give advice to current sufferers, one woman in a study of recovery by Rorty et al. (1993) expressed the sentiments of many participants in her reply: 'Don't give up. The path will take you in all different directions but it's worth it. Feel the feelings and expect to slip. No matter how long it takes you're better off in recovery than you are in the throes of bulimia.'

# Patient attitudes toward eating disorders

Two recent qualitative studies investigated patients' opinions about anorexia nervosa (Serpell et al., 1999) and bulimia nervosa (Brooks et al., 1998). The aim of the Serpell et al. (1999) study was to examine the attitudes of patients with anorexia nervosa toward their disorder. Eighteen individuals were asked to write two letters to their anorexia nervosa, one addressing the disorder as a friend and the other addressing it as an enemy. A coding scheme was devised to group recurrent themes expressed in the letters. The results demonstrated six common pro-themes which expressed patients' views on the perceived benefits of anorexia nervosa and three common anti-themes describing the perceived costs of the disorder. The most commonly expressed benefit of anorexia nervosa was its ability to help the patient feel safe, looked after and protected (the guardian theme). In this regard, the disorder was viewed as a dependable and consistent presence in the patient's life. In addition, patients saw their disorder as a friend which helped them to feel attractive and more appealing to men (the attractiveness theme); more self-confident in social relationships (the confidence theme) and special or even superior to others (difference theme). Finally, anorexia nervosa helped the patient by giving direction and structure to her life (control theme) and by allowing her to avoid distressing emotions, thoughts or events which she felt unable to cope with (avoid theme).

Patients also used three common anti-themes in their letters. One perceived cost of the disorder was the time and energy taken up by constant thoughts of food (food theme). A second perceived cost was the loss of friends and damage to personal relationship (social theme). Finally, many gave powerful descriptions of how anorexia nervosa had taken over their lives. They viewed the disorder as a force which stifled and depersonalized them (take-over theme). These letters reveal the great value which patients with anorexia nervosa attach to their disorder. They also offer possible explanations for resistance to offers of help. In addition, patients' views on perceived costs provide hints regarding potential motivational factors for recovery.

The Brooks *et al.* (1998) study employed semi-structured interviews with patients diagnosed with bulimia nervosa. The content of these interviews was explored using discourse analysis, an approach which analyzes the use of language in constructing views of the world and of oneself. The authors employed discourse analysis to investigate the ways in which patients with bulimia nervosa constructed their disorder. Five dominant views (repertoires) of bulimia nervosa resulted. In the first repertoire, bulimia nervosa was constructed as a thing which victimized and debilitated the patient, rendering her powerless. The second repertoire constructed bulimia nervosa as an act of self-inflicted punishment on the body for indulging in appetites. In the third repertoire, women were viewed as victims of social stereotypes; the thin, perfectly shaped stereotype of female beauty was seen as oppressive and disempowering, resulting in desperate measures to achieve the cultural ideal. A fourth repertoire depicted bulimia nervosa as a personality trait, a flaw in the individual which the patients usually related to lack of willpower or self-control. Marginalization of both the disorder and the patient herself constituted the fifth repertoire. The majority of patients constructed bulimia nervosa as abnormal and revolting and themselves as alien outsiders. These views underscore the importance of considering the sociocultural context and its disempowering impact on those who develop eating disorders.

# Patient views on factors which promote or sabotage recovery

In recent years, several authors (Hsu *et al.*, 1992; Rorty *et al.*, 1993; Yager *et al.*, 1989) have commented on how little attention has focussed on the patient's subjective experience of factors which have helped or hindered her efforts to recover. In a national magazine survey of 641 women with eating disorders, Yager *et al.* (1989) found little patient support for the efficacy of individual, behavioral, nutritional or group therapies. Caregivers selected as 'experts' in the treatment of eating disorders were rated as more efficacious than others. Hsu *et al.* (1992) asked six patients to describe their experience of recovery 20 years after the onset of their disorder. Several factors were identified as important to the recovery process. These included:

- personality strength; exercising personal willpower in a conscious determination to get well
- getting out of an abusive environment
- readiness to change and a feeling of being 'fed up' with the disorder
- being unconditionally accepted and understood by one's therapists.

In an investigation by Rorty *et al.* (1993), 40 women who were recovered from bulimia nervosa for one year or more were interviewed regarding factors they believed to be related to their recovery. The majority of the participants were motivated to recover by a desire for a better life or weariness of having their lives dominated by the disorder. Many also feared negative medical, social or professional consequences. Factors which the women highlighted as essential to recovery were empathic understanding and respect for the patient as a whole person. These qualities were viewed as important in all relationships including those with therapists, other patients, and significant others. Taking the disordered eating seriously while focussing on underlying causes was viewed as important. Factors seen as harmful to the recovery process included conceptualizing the disorder as a mere constellation of symptoms and active sabotage by others. With regard to the latter, many portrayed their parents as engaging in behaviors which were actively harmful to recovery. These behaviors included blaming the patient for her disorder, undermining her efforts to get help, providing insufficient emotional support and acts of direct sabotage such as deliberately buying tempting foods. Finally, support groups of various kinds, including those with a spiritual focus, were viewed as important components of the healing process.

Rose (personal communication, 1999) identified several factors which promoted her recovery, including medication to bring her depression under control first, attending a support group, an agreement with her family physician not to be informed of her weight and internet contacts with other sufferers who were non-judgmental and truly understood her situation. Factors which were not helpful and promoted relapse were hospitalization on a psychiatric unit (in contrast to an eating disorder clinic), being treated by professionals who were not knowledgeable about eating disorders (she found it too easy to deceive these individuals and thus maintain her self-starvation and laxative abuse) and the unavailability of individual psychotherapy and inadequate preparation for release at the treatment center.

Clearly, patients have much to teach us about what stimulates initiation of the recovery process, factors which promote recovery and circumstances which serve to sabotage it. What is also apparent is the wide variation in experience and the importance of understanding the divergent paths which individuals take on the road to recovery.

# Impact on function

The impact of an eating disorder on the individual's daily life can be pervasive. To varying degrees, school and work performance are compromised, daily activities are altered and relationships are deeply affected.

# Work and school performance

It takes a tremendous amount of energy and perseverance to maintain self-starvation and cope with the chaotic cycles of bingeing and purging. Over the course of the disorder, students find it increasingly difficult to concentrate on their studies. In most cases, this is not a result of an intrinsic lack of motivation; rather, most sufferers are very driven and achievement-oriented. In fact, being thin is viewed as a significant personal accomplishment, making it harder for the patient to give it up. Concentration is diminished due to fatigue related to malnutrition and intrusive thoughts about food and weight. Where there is extreme emaciation and malnourishment, the patient may also have difficulty concentrating on normal conversation, making it hard to benefit from psychotherapy. In bulimia nervosa, urges to binge and/or purge and emotional turmoil hamper the patient's ability to focus on a task. Eventually the combined effects of malnutrition and emotional distress can affect academic performance. It may be necessary to take extended periods of time away from school (i.e. during hospitalizations), a situation which can significantly alter academic plans and career direction. Some people are confused by this situation because it does not fit with the perfectionism and high self-expectations of the patient. For many sufferers, however, thinness becomes the ultimate accomplishment. Little pride may be felt or expressed regarding other achievements, talents or positive personal qualities.

In the workplace, most patients are viewed as diligent and conscientious. Some sufferers even describe themselves as workaholics, claiming that the busyness distracts them from thoughts of food and prevents them from eating. In addition, the frantic pace and crowded schedules serve to keep uncomfortable feelings at a distance. The stress of overwork, combined with biological and emotional stressors, can lead to a potentially volatile situation. Irritability, difficulty adapting to change and tendency to isolate may alienate the patient and create conflicts with co-workers and bosses.

Finally, patients also make frequent references to the inner voices which frustrate their abilities to concentrate, relax and maintain a positive self-concept. One patient (Thompson, 1996) explained her voices from within as a constant negative dialogue in her head; a source of torment from the time she wakes up until she falls asleep. Other patients have referred to this as their 'anorexic voice' or their 'bulimic monster'; some even have a name for her. The individual's sense of self-esteem and ability to function are seriously compromised by an inner voice which tells her she is worthless, disgusting and weak.

# Effects of the eating disorder on relationships

Eating disorders can have a profound impact on social, familial and intimate relationships.

In advanced stages, social isolation from peers is common in both anorexia nervosa and bulimia nervosa. Patients begin to eat alone and may withdraw from activities. Especially anxiety-provoking are social events which involve food, including eating at restaurants, parties and invitations to dinner. Patients become adept at making excuses to avoid confrontations about their eating habits. In addition, the initial attention gained from losing weight may now be very threatening, particularly for emaciated patients. Peers become frightened and don't know how to act. Unwanted stares, feelings of being avoided and comments about weight exacerbate self-consciousness, leading to further isolation.

Social isolation can also be the result of a sense of personal inferiority and an attempt to keep anger and hurt feelings buried. The dilemma becomes one of trying to maintain approval and acceptance in relationships when confronted by one's own feelings of rage, betrayal or fear. At the outset, most patients with eating disorders see no place for these emotions in interpersonal relationships. Fearing reprisals from being assertive, many continue to behave in compassionate and supportive ways even with those who have deeply hurt them.

Relationships within the family are also deeply affected. The patient may isolate herself by eating alone and withdrawing from family outings. She may spend inordinate amounts of time alone in her room to avoid contact. Within the relative safety of the family, some patients become irritable and verbally abrasive. Others may lose control over their emotions completely. Most react to this behavior with shame and express guilt over what they are 'putting the family through'. The reactions of parents and sibling are diverse and may include anger and feeling betrayed by a child who was always 'such a good girl', frustration at the difficulty in understanding the dynamics of an eating disorder, fear of losing their daughter and guilt or self-blame. Others respond with disgust and rejection of the patient. This reaction can arise in connection to an abusive relationship or it may be due to misinformation and ignorance about the biological/psychological dynamics of eating disorders. Siblings express a variety of reactions including worries about the patient's health and anger toward her for creating stress in the family or, in the case of binge eating, for eating more than their share of food in the home. Unfortunately, negative reactions from family members, if not addressed, can heighten family stress, estrange the patient further and exacerbate the eating disorder.

Many sufferers function in the home by taking on the role of the 'super-responsible daughter'. Mather (1997) described her tendency to put the needs and wants of other family members before her own. In her spare time, she would clean the house, bake and take responsibility for the happiness of others. The recognition and praise she got for this became very important to her. In the author's experience, many patients try to take on the role of nurturer and caregiver in the family. They worry inordinately about the welfare of other family members and become very skilled at intuiting and responding to the needs of parents and siblings.

One important area of functioning which has received little attention in the literature is the impact of the eating disorder on the mother's relationship to her children. Lacey and Smith (1987) found that the prevalence of binge eating and vomiting among individuals with bulimia nervosa decreased sequentially during each trimester of the pregnancy. However, symptoms returned after delivery in two-thirds of the patients. In addition, a higher-than-expected rate of 'failure to thrive' was found among the infants. Similarly, some patients with anorexia nervosa claim that during pregnancy they are able to eat well-balanced, more nutritious meals because they believe that the nourishment is for the unborn child and not for themselves.

During pregnancy, adaptation to bodily changes such as enlarged breasts and hips and a protruding abdomen may be very stressful for those already uncomfortable with their bodies (Olmsted, 1992). Fears of being out of control may also be amplified during this period. According to Zerbe (1993), heightened concerns about identity, autonomy and personal adequacy may trigger a relapse and eating disorder symptoms may return or be exacerbated.

Concerns have also been expressed about restrictive feeding practices for infants and small children (Zerbe, 1993) and excessive worry about the child's food intake and weight (Woodside and Shekter-Wolfson, 1990). This concern is related to the mother's preoccupation with her own weight and fears that her child will become fat.

Since this chapter is concerned with the patient's perceptions, it is also important to point out that individuals who suffer with eating disorders often feel wrongly accused of putting their infants and young children on semi-starvation diets. They resent the assumption that current thinness or history of an eating disorder is evidence of an inability to care for their own children. Olmsted (1992) has underlined the importance of planning for the pregnant body through education, emotional support and close monitoring of the woman with an active eating disorder.

The author's experience has shown that as mothers, patients may also be very vigilant and anxious about their children's weight as they grow up. When the child is older, she may elicit a daughter's help in monitoring her own food intake or the two may go on a diet together. Finally, female children who witness their mother's body image disparagement, constant dieting, and/or compulsive exercising can be strongly influenced in terms of their own beliefs and behavior around food and weight.

Patients who experience a heightened sense of personal responsibility can have difficulty functioning in close, intimate relationships. Their deep longings for approval exist alongside fears of rejection and strong needs for personal control. Despite strong cravings to be held and nurtured, they often reject attempts to hug or touch them. As Hornbacher (1998) explained, the needs for contact are so great, the patient begins to fear or be ashamed of them. This reaction, combined with body shame, can contribute to physical and emotional distancing in relationships.

Finally, the presence of an eating disorder can significantly affect sexual functioning. According to Zerbe (1993), patients who are affected by anorexia nervosa report low levels of sexual interest and activity whereas those with bulimia nervosa tend to be more sexually active. Patients report feeling out of control, guilty for seeking pleasure and ambivalent about their own sexual desires, fantasies and behavior. The voice of Karen (aged 20) demonstrates these conflictual feelings: 'I'm just not interested in sex any more. I want to be but I'm not. I feel so insecure about my body. I want physical affection but just the thought of having sex makes me feel gross and taken over, sort of.'

Peters and Fallon (1994) reported that patients also express difficulty establishing trust and self-confidence in sexual relationships, particularly those who have been sexually or physically abused. The authors presented the results of an interview study of women recovering from bulimia nervosa. The participants expressed a great deal of confusion about their sexuality and fears of being vulnerable. Some used their bodies to elicit male approval and had difficulty relating to men who treated them well. As Zerbe (1993) has noted, however, some patients with bulimia nervosa completely stifle their sexuality as a way of coping with grief, loss and fears of abandonment.

# Expectations of the clinician

As indicated earlier in this chapter, many individuals have come to expect and fear negative reactions from clinicians. Patients have felt the blame ('be sensible'; 'you're not trying'; 'this is a choice, you know') and contempt of practitioners who accused them of being manipulative and deceitful. They have resented being silenced and punished. Condescending attitudes on the part of clinicians have often resulted in hopelessness and aversion to treatment. It is interesting to note that while most patients detest tube-feeding, required food intakes and restricted access to bathrooms and exercise, they often express some understanding of the need for these interventions under extreme circumstances. What they do not accept are restrictions which isolate them from family and friends. These restrictions plus the cold administration of the above-mentioned procedures can meet with resentment and retaliation, especially when the patient is not allowed to voice her fear, anger and need for support. As Ostroff (Hall and Ostroff, 1999) has explained, individuals suffering with eating disorders need, above all, to be treated with respect, compassion and 'unflagging support'. Kindness and optimism not only keeps the patient in therapy, it teaches her to be gentle and compassionate with herself.

No discussion of patient expectations is complete without addressing the fact that some patients (especially those in the throes of anorexia nervosa) do not want our help. They are explicit about their desire to be left alone. In addition, many individuals request help with their emotional distress and its impact on school, work and relationships but they want to recover without gaining weight. Their steadfast belief is that one can continue to diet and still overcome the psychological torment of self-starvation and/or eliminate the cycles of bingeing and purging. These issues are discussed in detail in the chapter on management and finding common ground.

What is it that individuals who struggle with eating disorders expect from clinicians and the treatment programs they offer? The following list summarizes the views of patients represented in the literature and in the author's clinical practice:

- approaches which focus on both the normalization of eating patterns and underlying emotional issues and low self-esteem
- approaches which empower the patient (i.e. through providing accurate information and involving her in decisions regarding the treatment process)

- approaches which address the whole person, honoring the unique background, experiences and emotional needs of the sufferer
- approaches which demonstrate a knowledge of the emotional and cognitive dynamics (the 'inner voice') of eating disorders
- approaches which do not rely solely on drugs. Patients need genuine human contact and relationships
- approaches which offer alternate coping strategies when self-starvation and bingeing/purging behaviors are taken away
- approaches which offer emotional and spiritual healing.

Since outpatient treatment of individuals with eating disorders often involves a team of professionals (physician, psychotherapist, dietitian, family therapist) and non-professional supports (i.e. support groups), it is helpful to note the specific expectations patients have with regard to their participation in her recovery.

Patients want a family physician who is compassionate, respectful and knowledgeable with regard to the medical consequences of self-starvation, bingeing and purging. They expect that the physician will explain the medical risks of their disorder and the side effects of any prescribed drugs in comprehensible terms. Since the physician is likely to be the one recording weight and vital signs, they need him/her to be sensitive to their fears of weight gain and negative body image. Some patients benefit from not knowing their weight. In addition, patients need their physician and his/her staff to understand that comments like 'Oh, you've gained weight this week. Good for you!' or 'I can tell you're eating a lot more than before. Your face is getting fuller' are likely to be misinterpreted as 'You're getting fat' and therefore are not helpful. Finally, patients expect that their family physician will be willing to work in collaboration with other professionals involved in their care.

Individuals with anorexia nervosa or bulimia nervosa are also clear about the qualities they expect in a therapist whether this individual is a psychologist, psychiatrist, art therapist or social worker, etc. Patients are consistent about their need for a therapist who is warm, empathic and genuine. They want therapists who are knowledgeable about eating disorders, who approach them as unique individuals and who comprehend the 'inner eating-disorder voice' and how it can rule their lives. This person also needs to demonstrate a willingness to co-operate with other members of the outpatient team.

In their work with the dietitian, sufferers have frequently expressed a need to see someone whose nutritional counseling goes beyond an explanation of The Food Pyramid US (Canada's Food Guide). Those who struggle with eating disorders feel that this approach fails to recognize their intense fears of weight gain and their need to take things slowly. In addition, patients expect their dietitian to individualize their treatment in a way that takes into account their idiosyncratic relationship to food. This includes being vegetarian or vegan by choice, cultural issues around food, food phobias, ritualistic eating and viewing food as the enemy.

With regards to the family therapist, patients also expect collaboration and a warm, compassionate approach. Some individuals enter family therapy with the fear that the entire process will focus on the patient as the problem. Patients have expressed fears of being emotionally annihilated or devoured by other members of the family as a result of personal disclosure. They fear a total loss of control over their own lives, a fear which often exists alongside tremendous shame and guilt for what she has 'put the family through'. The patient needs the family therapist to understand this. One patient who was extremely protective of her parents became very resistant in family therapy sessions. While the hour focussed on the young woman's eating disorder and how it affected family members, her resistance was as much related to the fact that she was the keeper of the mother's secret marital affair as it was to relinquishing her bulimia. Another adolescent's resentment of family therapy was related to her feeling that she was being pressured to give up the very behaviors (dieting, exercising) she has originally been cajoled into by her parents. Patients expect the family therapist to be aware of and sensitive to the other forces operating in their lives. Many welcome family therapy as a vehicle for expressing feelings to parents and siblings, for relieving them of felt responsibility for the welfare of the entire family and finally as a place where they can enlist the therapist's assistance in explaining the dynamics of their eating disorder and how it involves all family members.

Patient expectations for support groups have also been expressed. Most state a preference for smaller groups of individuals from the same age bracket. Beyond learning psychoeducational tools for recovery, individuals with eating disorders want groups which instill optimism and hope. The common experiences and testimonials of others serve to do this. Patients often express a need to share their thoughts, questions and feelings with someone who 'truly understands' their struggle.

In summary, patients with eating disorders are often very clear about what they need and expect from practitioners. Many have read extensively on the subject themselves; others have been through countless attempts at treatment and need to have their voices heard in terms of what was helpful and what was not helpful to them as an individual.

This chapter has focused on the patient's voice in order to enhance our understanding of anorexia nervosa and bulimia nervosa. An appreciation of the patient's ideas and opinions, emotional experiences, expectations of the clinician, and ability to cope with their daily life fosters the development of common ground between patient and clinician and is thus fundamental to the patient-centered approach. Clearly, more qualitative studies are required. Patients have much to teach us about the etiology, symptoms, impact and healing factors related to eating disorders.

# References

Brooks A, LeCouteur A and Hepworth J (1998) Accounts of experiences of bulimia: a discourse analytic study. *Int J Eating Disord.* 24: 193–205.

Fodor V (1997) *Desperately Seeking Self.* Gurze Books, Carlsbad, CA.

Hall L and Cohn L (1999) *Bulimia: a guide to recovery.* Gurze Books, Carlsbad, CA.

Hall L and Ostroff M (1999) *Anorexia Nervosa: a guide to recovery.* Gurze Books, Carlsbad, CA.

Hornbacher M (1998) *Wasted.* Harper Collins, New York.

Hsu LKG, Crisp AH and Callender JS (1992) Recovery in anorexia nervosa: the patient's perspective. *Int J Eat Disord.* 11: 341–50.

Lacey H and Smith G (1987) Bulimia nervosa: the impact of pregnancy on mother and baby. *Br J Psychiatry.* 150: 777–81.

MacLeod S (1981) *The Art of Starvation.* Virago, London, UK.

Mather SA (1997) *Leaving Food Behind.* Mather Publication for Growth and Wellness, Inc, Nepean, ON, Canada.

Medina A (1998) Tips for doctors. Available at www.something-fishy.org (website on eating disorders)

Normandi CE and Roark L (1998) *It's Not About Food.* Penguin Putnam Inc, New York.

Olmsted MP (1992, October) Planning for the pregnant body. *Nat Eat Disord Inform Centre Bull.* 7(4): 1–2.

Peters L and Fallon P (1994) The journey of recovery: dimensions of change. In: P Fallon, MA Katzman and SC Wooley (eds) *Femininst Perspectives on Eating Disorders.* Guilford Press, New York.

Rorty M, Yager J and Rossotto E (1993) Why and how do women recover from bulimia nervosa?: the subjective appraisals of 40 women recovered for a year or more. *Int J Eat Disord.* 14: 249–60.

Serpell L, Treasure J, Teasdale J and Sullivan V (1999) Anorexia nervosa: friend or foe? *Int J Eat Disord.* 25: 177–86.

Thompson C (1996) The voices from within. Available at www.mirror-mirror.org (website for eating disorders).

Vitousek KB, Daly T and Heiser C (1991) Reconstructing the internal world of the eating-disordered individual: overcoming denial and distortion in self-report. *Int J Eat Disord.* 10: 647–66.

Woodside DB and Shekter-Wolfson LF (1990) Parenting by parents with anorexia nervosa and bulimia nervosa. *Int J Eat Disord.* 9: 303–9.

Yager J, Landsverk J and Edelstein CK (1989) Help-seeking and satisfaction with care in 641 women with eating disorders. *J Nerv Ment Dis.* 177: 632–7.

Zerbe KJ (1993) *The Body Betrayed: women, eating disorders and treatment.* American Psychiatric Press, Washington DC.

# 4

# Understanding the whole person: Rose's story

A patient-centered view of eating disorders requires an approach which focuses on the individual's unique story in the development of and recovery from anorexia nervosa or bulimia nervosa. Understanding the whole person requires an appreciation of the circumstances within which the eating disorder developed, and sensitivity to the multiple factors which influence the patient's illness experience (Stewart *et al.*, 1995). This includes the individual's age and developmental stage at onset, the corresponding point in the family lifecycle and personal experiences including trauma, friendship networks, school, employment, religion and cultural traditions and beliefs. In the patient-centered approach, the clinician needs to be familiar with the patient's ethnicity and membership in cultural subgroups related to social class, gender, sexual preference, marital status, educational level and occupation (Stewart *et al.*, 1995). The norms and values attached to these subgroups affect how the patient and her family conceptualize the eating disorder in terms of causation, treatment options, reactions to emotional, behavioral and physical symptoms and expectations of the healthcare system. Therefore, an understanding of the whole person must also include an appreciation of the impact of the eating disorder on social, familial and personal aspects of the individual's life and the ways in which these may have maintained the eating disorder across the lifespan.

Rose's story is an example of how these diverse factors intersect to impact on the life of a child, adolescent and young woman. In her own voice, Rose tells of the experiences and circumstances which contributed to the development of her eating disorder and served to exacerbate existing symptoms. She describes her reactions to treatment approaches and the factors which she considers to be most influential in her recovery. Her story is told with candor, insight and courage. It holds a powerful message for both professionals and loved ones about the importance of taking the whole person into account in order to understand and support the healing of those who suffer from eating disorders.

# Rose's story

I am a 36-year-old married woman and I have suffered from an eating disorder for over half my life. It came in many forms. Anorexia was the predominant and consistent disorder, although I went through a variety of bulimic episodes. I believe there are many misconceptions regarding eating disorders. I'm writing my story in the hope of shedding light on eating disorders, and the individuals who suffer from them. In order for me to fully explain the precursors to an eating disorder and how it develops and manifests itself in an individual, I need to share with the reader intimate and personal events in my life. Therefore, after a lot of consideration I have decided to write under a pen name, not out of shame or embarrassment, but to protect the anonymity of my family and myself.

Throughout this chapter I will be describing events in my life. Since family is a large part of everyone's life, I do speak of my family. When I refer to my family I speak of things that affected my eating disorder and myself. Therefore, the views that I express here are my own subjective perception of events. Other family members may have a different perception of the events and may not share these views.

The first time I realized that I was battling an eating disorder was after watching a television program where a person experienced with eating disorders was being interviewed. She explained the mind-set of someone with an eating disorder. She described perfectly the way I felt and the way I thought. I realized that what I had was called an 'eating disorder'. Until then I knew that there was something wrong with me, but I didn't know what it was. I felt relief. I wasn't crazy. There was a name for what I was going through. Although I now understand that I was still in denial. I began to visit eating disorder chat groups and news groups on the Internet. I met people like myself, going through the same emotions and confusion I was. It was wonderful and horrible at the same time. I learned about treatment, successes and failures. I received support and love, but most of all I received understanding. For the first time I accepted the fact that I had an eating disorder, although this acceptance was mixed with denial.

Some groups had strict rules about not giving details of what one had done to perpetuate an eating disorder, some didn't. Being deep within my eating disorder, I visited those that didn't have rules and scrolled for tips. This included tips on losing more weight, using tactics I hadn't thought of and using products I wasn't aware of, all the while accepting the fact that I did indeed have an eating disorder, but at the same time doing anything I could to perpetuate it. I was not alone in this, which is why the rules of not discussing numerical weight or dieting tricks were in place.

When I did finally admit to those close to me that I was dealing with an eating disorder I had a strong support system in place. My family physician was wonderful. She had me in her office at least once a week, not only to get weighed and monitor my health but also to talk about my feelings and how I was dealing with my impending admittance to an eating-disorders clinic. My psychiatrist was an incredible support for me. I would see her twice a week and more often if I needed. I wasn't ready to admit that my personal issues were at all related to my eating disorder, but she was patient with me. I spent a lot of time on the Internet, in electronic support groups. Many of the people there had been to treatment and quelled some of my fears. I was on the Internet everyday as this was my greatest source of support. These people understood; many had been at the place where I was at the time.

# The development of my eating disorder: early influences

My eating disorder first presented itself when I was around the age of 13. I started to develop and gain weight. Until that time I was very thin. My family took great pride in the fact that I was so thin, so for me to gain weight meant that I was disappointing them. I started to restrict my food intake and take my mother's diet pills. I found an incredible amount of personal satisfaction in being able to manipulate my weight. I felt in control. Everything in my life was out of control but through my eating disorder I could control the one thing that was mine and mine alone: **my body**. I was actually able to hide my eating disorder for many years due to the fact that I was so thin as a child. My parents had no idea, but my friends did become suspicious in my late teens. I was a ballet dancer, so being very thin was expected and encouraged. I learned 'diet tricks' from the older dancers. Coffee and cigarettes soon became my staple diet. My mother and grandmother were always on some sort of a diet, or 'eating program' as my grandmother would refer to it. I learned that it was normal to diet; everyone did it. My mother, my grandmother, my ballet friends. I was just doing it for different reasons, but the reasons were irrelevant. I was dieting like everyone else.

I was complimented within my family for losing weight, for controlling my weight, until I would refuse to bend from my stringent eating rules. My parents would react with anger towards my various diets and increasingly bizarre eating habits. They expressed concern not at my weight loss, but at my eating habits. They would get angry at my unbending insistence to follow my chosen eating style with extreme precision. An example of bizarre or ritualistic eating habit would be the way I ate an orange or grapefruit. I would peel the orange and separate it; I would then take one section, remove the skin and eat the kernels inside one by one. The section would take about half an hour to eat. I would eat approximately two slices in a sitting and the whole orange would last me all day. The thought process behind this was that it took a long time to eat, so I would feel like I had been eating forever and therefore I was full. There were ways to trick my mind into making me feel full and satiated. I would also eat soda crackers in a ritualistic fashion. I looked at the box and calculated how many calories four crackers had. I then knew I could eat four crackers. I would take one cracker and split it with extreme precision using my teeth, eating the top half first, taking tiny bites and chewing only with my front teeth. I would eat the bottom half the same way, only in tiny bites and chewing with my front teeth. I would never finish the bottom half of the cracker, which I gave to my dog. In actuality, I didn't even eat a whole cracker. This was done in such a trance like state that I didn't even realize that I was giving most of my cracker to my dog.

In high school, my parents and friends would ask what was wrong; was I dieting, what was I doing? I, of course, denied it all. In university, my friends confronted me and said that they suspected that I had anorexia and that I needed medical attention. I never did seek medical attention; I thought they were overreacting. In my 20s and 30s no one said anything; they would just whisper behind my back.

I was trying to achieve perfection, control and praise. It started with my body developing. My hips expanded, my breasts started to get larger. This happened quite quickly. It made me feel uncomfortable with my body. I wanted to be thin and 'sexless' like I was when I was younger. In ballet, a boy-like figure is ideal. I didn't like the attention my developing body brought. I was complemented on my developing figure; this made me feel very uncomfortable. It made me very self-conscious when my mother would say that she envied my figure, my rounded hips and full breasts. She would describe in detail how thin she was before she had children. In addition, my mother often asked me my weight and compared it with her own weight. I interpreted this as my body not belonging to me, it was just one more thing that was someone else's property. By dieting, I discovered control for the first time in my life. I could control the size and shape of my body.

My parents seemed pleased that I was a thin child who could eat anything and not gain weight. This started to change when my body started to develop. I wanted to please them, to not lose their love and praise. People at school would envy me that I could eat anything and not gain weight. Once again, friends were envious. I saw my mother's friends compliment her on her weight loss. I think that is where I got the idea that weight control equals praise. A large part of keeping thin was to keep myself from developing into a sexual being and avoid any attention that comes with one developing. I was praised by my ballet teacher, and made an example of for the other students. In ballet, a thin body is an ideal body. I had it, and others envied me for it. I would get praise.

# Diagnosis and denial

It wasn't until my 20s that I was actually diagnosed with an eating disorder. I was admitted to hospital for a severe electrolyte imbalance, due to laxative abuse. Until that time I was able to hide my eating disorder from everyone. Once my eating disorder was out in the open, I still denied that I had any sort of a problem. After being stabilized I was released. I started using laxatives again, and once again I ended up in the hospital with an electrolyte imbalance. Once released and stabilized the second time I didn't touch laxatives again. Since I gained weight not using the laxatives, I started restricting. I was restricting before, but without the laxatives I became extremely strict regarding my food intake. This now became a cat-and-mouse game with my doctor. I denied restricting. The EKG showed arrhythmia, but I played stupid. I was determined that they (the doctors) wouldn't find out what I was doing. I was seeing a dietitian at the time, and filled out my daily intake sheet like a grocery list. Anything to make her happy and not tell my doctor.

At the time of my diagnosis I was very angry with everyone. As far as I was concerned, I didn't have a problem, I just wanted to maintain my weight. Secretly I still wanted to lose more; I did. At the time I didn't know why it was so important to me to keep losing weight. If anyone said it was a way of not dealing with my problems, I would say, 'What problems? I don't have any problems. I'm just a useless, horrid being that doesn't deserve to take up space on this earth'. I didn't view that as a problem. To me a problem was running out of gas, or not being able to get to the post office on time. I interpreted my lack of self-worth as a foregone conclusion; something that I had no control over and no power to change. I didn't even realize that I had no self-worth until much later in my therapy. I just knew that I was a bad person. I didn't know why, or how it had happened. I explained it to myself that I was just born that way.

The insistence of my doctors that I was at a critical stage only reinforced my determination to maintain my eating disorder at any cost, including losing friends, family, jeopardizing my marriage and even death. The more everyone pushed me to get help, the more I felt that I was succeeding. When people would tell me that I was incredibly thin, I felt like I was on a mental and emotional high. Since I had been severely depressed for years, this high was a welcome change. I think that was one of the reasons that I fought treatment so voraciously. The most important reason was that the eating disorder was the one thing in my life I believed that I did well. I accomplished what others couldn't. It also fed my desire to disappear, to be invisible, to not take up space. Treatment meant that all of this would be taken away from me. I had fought so hard to get to where I was, and now people who had no idea of how I felt and what my eating disorder did for me just wanted me to give it up.

In my mind I idealized my eating disorder. When it came time to give it up, I forgot all the horror that it had brought with it. I still have a hard time seeing my eating disorder as something I did to cope with my life. I viewed it as a separate entity, and yet an integral part of myself. I speak of it as if it almost were a separate being within me, which coincides with my view of myself. I see the person who went through terrible trauma and had a dysfunctional family as separate from myself. I dissociate myself from that person, perhaps because I'm not ready to face the pain that will inevitably come with accepting that we are one and the same.

# Symptoms

It was not until my 20s that I personally noticed any physical symptoms resultng from my ongoing eating disorder. The symptoms would depend on the form which my eating disorder took. They varied during purging and restricting stages. Other variants included age, stress level and environment. The earliest, most common and most consistent symptom regardless of which weight-control method I was using was physical weakness. It would manifest itself as extreme tiredness and mental exhaustion, although I was able to perform physically. The later symptoms depended on whether I was purging or restricting.

Table 4.1 lists the early and latter symptoms and signs of both the bulimic and anorexic phases of my eating disorder. Most of these symptoms are examples of those discussed in Chapter 1. They illustrate one individual's unique experiences with her body's physiological reactions to an eating disorder.

Although the symptoms appear to be quite debilitating, I was able to carry on with my everyday life effectively and efficiently. Despite my constant feeling of weakness, I seemed to have an abundance of energy. This enabled me to hide my eating disorder so well and for so long. During my teen years, the symptoms were often mistaken for normal developmental changes, so it was quite easy to keep my disorder hidden. Once older, it became more difficult to hide my symptoms, and to perform at an optimum level at work. Amongst adults, people would question the changes in moods and physical appearance, yet I was able to put people off with explanations that they would accept. For example, I would tell people that I had the flu, irritable bowel syndrome or simply loss of appetite.

# Contributing factors: personality traits and personal values

There are several contributing factors that I've become aware of over the course of my eating disorder and therapy (these seem to be quite common among my

**Table 4.1:** Early and later symptoms of Rose's anorectic/bulimic phases

| Eating disorder | Early symptoms/signs | Later symptoms/signs |
| --- | --- | --- |
| **Purging (laxative abuse/ self-induced vomiting)** | Weakness<br>Dizziness<br>Dehydration<br>Sore throat<br>Trips to bathroom after meal, or taking showers | Heart palpitations<br>Electrolyte imbalance<br>Fainting<br>Inability to control bowels<br>Burning in esophagus |
| | Restricting during the day and eating at night | Inability to self-induce vomiting |
| | Spending money on laxatives or herbal preparations | Spending large amounts of money on laxatives<br>Traveling to different drug stores to purchase laxatives with the fear that the sales people will recognize you |
| **Restriction of food intake** | Weakness | Fainting |
| | Dizziness | Insomnia |
| | Fainting | Extreme weight loss |
| | Extreme hunger pains | Listlessness |
| | Eliminating specific foods (i.e. meat) | Depression |
| | Starting to exhibit ritualistic eating behaviors | Loss of interest in everything |
| | Avoiding meal times | Dehydration<br>Heart palpitations<br>Refusing to participate in meal times<br>Fear of restaurants<br>Ritualistic eating |

friends with eating disorders): family issues, trauma, and personality. Personality traits play a large part. I'm a perfectionist, have strict rules and guidelines for myself which don't apply to others. I wouldn't dream of imposing them on anyone else, or expect anyone else to abide by them. They are only for me. This perfectionism can become debilitating at times. The knowledge that I'm not perfect (how could I be when I'm such a loser) and the overwhelming desire to be perfect and perform perfectly is immobilizing. With this in mind, how is it possible for me to do a perfect job. This result is what I call 'perfection paralysis'. I felt paralyzed by the fear of not being able to do a perfect job and, therefore, I was terrified to even make an attempt. This leads me to another personality trait: low self-esteem. The reason why I felt the need to be perfect was that I had no self-esteem. To this day, I am working on feeling like a good person deserving of kindness and compassion. I felt, and somewhat still feel, like the most horrible monster of a person ever born, at times not deserving of being referred to as a human being. Every day I battle these feelings; feelings of being undeserving of love and kindness, feelings of being the ugliest person to walk the face of this earth. In public, I become afraid that people can see the 'real' *me*, the me that I see and not the person I portray. I become very self-conscious of any person looking at me and I project my own thoughts of myself onto them. Due to my issues with self-esteem and perfectionism, I'm also a 'people pleaser'. Feeling unworthy of anything, one way for me to feel worthy of people's kindness is to do whatever would make them happy or to please them. This applies to my parents, grandparents, friends and co-workers, anyone and everyone. I put other people's needs, wants and desires before my own, even at detriment to myself. In fact, the more I sacrifice myself for others the better I felt about myself. I have always felt a 'badness' within myself, and by always doing for others and thinking of others, I felt that I was cleansing the evil from within myself. The more I suffered, the more I was cleansed. The eating disorder is a perfect example of sacrificing myself, of personal suffering as a way of personal cleansing. Bulimia is quite symbolic of this; you purge the food (which symbolizes the evil) and by this you perform a ritual cleansing of your self. Also, by restricting your food intake, you get hunger pains (at the start). To suffer through these, you feel somehow cleansed of the evil being symbolized by food.

I have found throughout my life that I've always suppressed my emotions. I didn't discover this until I started therapy. I would never let anyone see how I was feeling. To others, I seemed very happy, while on the inside I was in horrible emotional pain. In art therapy, I came upon the symbolic idea of wearing masks. I realized that I had many masks. My 'happy mask' was the one that I wore the most. I believe this was the reason that it was such a shock to all that I was actually depressed. I knew it to be true, yet I couldn't let anyone else know. To me that would have been a sign of weakness, of not being perfect. It was okay for others to be sad, have a bad day, to be in pain, to have depression, etc., but for me those rules did not apply. Anger, sadness and rage are the most difficult emotions for me. To this day I'm afraid that if I let those emotions loose I will not be able to control them. To me control is all-important. Control is everything; it is personal power. Our society looks at thin women as in control, powerful, successful. If overweight, they are perceived as and labeled 'out of control, lazy'. This was definitely not the cause or contributor of my eating disorder, but it was definitely a catalyst. It confirmed in my mind that my eating disorder made me powerful and in control. It confirmed in my mind that by not eating I was portraying the image of one in control of one's life. Although this could not have been farther from the truth, it was my perception of myself.

Being in recovery now, I'm still affected when I see very thin actors, models or average people. I desire once again to be thin, very thin, like I was at my worst. Knowing all that I know, and all that I've been through to get to where I am today, the desire still calls to me and it is a temptation I battle every day.

# Contributing factors: familial, sociocultural and traumatic experiences

In my own case, family conflicts, parenting my younger brothers, culture shock, abandonment, grief, loss, sexual assault and participation in sport, where a particular body type is preferred and encouraged, were predisposing factors that contributed to the perpetuation of my eating disorder.

The environment in which I grew up was a factor in the development of my eating disorder. I believe the manner in which my parents expressed their views contributed to this. I come from a family in which there are unresolved conflicts. Experiences during my early childhood, my parents' reactions to traumatic events in my life and their response to my eating disorder, made it difficult for me. I won't go into specific detail regarding family issues, but will give an overview. My perception was that my parents where constantly angry and under stress. I didn't know the source, but I assumed it was me. They had trouble with conflict resolution, and there was a lot of family conflict.

My paternal grandparents raised me from birth to four years of age, as my parents were still in university when I was born. Around the same time, I moved with my parents from Eastern Europe to Canada and my grandparents moved to Western Europe. Leaving my grandparents was a great loss to me, and resulted in a feeling of not belonging throughout my life. Fleeing our homeland was very dangerous, any mistake on my part could have endangered the lives of my entire family. I don't want to go into any detail here, but will say that it was a time of war in which a Communist country invaded the one in which we lived. This was very traumatic for me, and gave me no time to grieve for the loss of my grandparents. Once in Canada, none of us spoke English. My parents took classes and I first became exposed to the English language when I enrolled in school at the age of five. This was a very difficult time for me, as I felt very alone. Not only was there the issue of the language barrier, but also culture shock. I felt I had to be strong, as we were all going through this together. I believe that this was the point at which I started to develop my caretaker role. I am the oldest of three, with seven years between my middle sibling and myself, and nine years between my youngest sibling and myself. Being the oldest and a daughter it was my responsibility to help around the house and with the care of my younger siblings. Throughout my life I spent my summers with my grandparents, or they would come to Canada for the summer. Either way, I saw my grandparents each summer. I found myself trying to be perfect and exactly what everyone wanted. In fact, I really didn't know who I was until my late 20s. I was so afraid that either set of 'parents' would reject me that I did anything to please everyone.

I was raped at age 15. I will go into more detail on this and how it effected my eating disorder later. I tried to commit suicide twice at 15 years old. These were both related to the depression and the rape. At 18/19, I lived with my grandparents in Germany for seven months. At 19, my parents and siblings moved to Saudi Arabia and I remained in Canada alone. Once again, I felt a sense of abandonment. My paternal grandfather died shortly after my family moved. I was unable to attend the funeral. I still have many unresolved issues surrounding this traumatic event in my life. During my 20s I tried to commit suicide four times. This was a period in my life in which I struggled with deep depression and my eating disorder was at its worst.

The rape at age 15 was by a stranger. I didn't tell anyone immediately. I was severely traumatized. I told my girlfriend and swore her to secrecy. I told a school guidance counselor who questioned the validity of my story. It was several months before I told my parents. I tried very hard to distance myself from my emotions. I didn't want anyone to know what had happened to me, so I pretended I was fine. At times, I pretended so well I would begin to question my own perceptions and instincts. I acted out my shame, anger and fear on my own body. My body became my enemy. Food became the catalyst which enabled me to punish my body. At this time I also began cutting myself. I felt my body was dirty. This would later lead to laxative abuse in a symbolic cleansing ritual. By not eating I was able to make my body smaller, to take up less space. I felt I had no control over my emotions, so I controlled my food and my body. This gave me a false sense of control over my life. I lost the ability to trust. This I transferred to myself as well. I didn't trust my emotions, I didn't trust my body. Therefore, when I looked in the mirror, I didn't trust my eyes. Eventually, I would begin to see the monster that I felt I was. I couldn't express anger or rage against anyone else, so I expressed my feelings against myself. The rape confirmed in my mind that I was a bad person and didn't deserve to take up space.

At 18, I was raped in the dorm of my university. It was date rape, but at the time, that expression didn't exist. Because of that, I blamed myself even more than I did with the first rape. Thoughts of 'I should have' and 'could have' plagued my mind. In that sense, this rape was more traumatic for me. It heightened my self-blame and self-loathing. My responses to the rape were numerous and included flashbacks, dreams, nightmares, denial, detachment, bursts of anger and rage, crying bouts, dysfunctional sleep patterns, difficulty concentrating, anxiety, depression, emotional turmoil, shame, emotional numbness and a sense of a foreshortened future.

I began bingeing and purging. I ate because it had a numbing effect and I purged because to me the food was still evil, so I had to get it out of my body.

From that time onward, my eating disorder was constant. There were no rest periods in between. It was an unending assault on my body.

I now understand that my suicide attempts were multifaceted, the primary cause being severe depression. I felt that it was the only escape for me. At the time I saw no other means of solving my problems or dealing with my life. Actually, I didn't deal with my problems. I would bury them, but they did surface. The suicide attempts in my teens were a cry for help. I also thought that if I did succeed in killing myself then everyone would be better off, especially my family. I saw myself as a problem to my family. I was the bad one, I was the one causing problems. The battle in my head, of wondering what it was that I did that made me such a bad person and wondering why my parents were so angry with me, was unbearable. As for emotions related to my eating disorder, I just wanted them to stop. I saw only two possibilities for this to happen: 1) tell someone, which would result in getting help, which would result in having to gain weight – this was not an option for me; 2) kill myself, and stop the pain inside me, and the pain I was causing my family. I couldn't stand what I was doing to my family.

My personal feelings surrounding my suicide attempts at 15 are really non-existent. At the time I didn't see another possible solution. I feel the same about the attempts in my 20s.

I portrayed such a happy and in-control person; it came as a shock. My family reacted with shock, confusion, hurt and anger. As the attempts became more frequent, the shock wore off and all that was left was confusion, hurt and anger. My husband was worried and scared. As time went on and the attempts continued, he became hurt. After many years, his anger surfaced once he was sure that I was not in danger any more.

# Treatment

I was hospitalized numerous times. One facility was the psychiatric unit of a general hospital to which I was admitted numerous times. The other was a treatment center specifically directed at eating disorders. My admissions to the psychiatric unit were for various reasons, including depression, suicide attempts and my eating disorder. The main purpose of the unit was to treat depression and secure personal safety before discharge. There was a significant emphasis on therapy, but little concentration on the eating disorder itself. As this was a hospital and not a treatment center, once a person was deemed safe, they were discharged. I was able to select my own meals off the menu and had no supervision during meals. I was, therefore, able to perpetuate my disorder while in the hospital.

The treatment center was quite different. First, I must say that there was a long waiting list. All the treatment centers that my family physician contacted had waiting lists of six months to a year. I agreed to have her contact the centers and add my name to the waiting list, knowing that at this point I needed specialized help. It took six months before I got a call that they would have a bed available for me. I had to make the decision on the spot, and agree to be there in one week, or my bed would be given to someone else. I was warned in the literature forwarded to me that this would be the case, but I was not prepared. The day came for my husband to drive me to the center. I begged him not to take me there, not to leave me there. I promised that I would eat, I promised anything I could think of, just so that he would take me back home.

My recollection of that day is not as clear as my husband's. He remembers it as if it was yesterday, and becomes overwhelmed with emotion at the thought of that day. I remember clearly walking on to the eating disorders unit, seeing the other people on the floor and thinking that I definitely didn't belong there. I looked at everyone and they were so thin, it solidified the thought in my mind that I didn't have a problem. I was not nearly as thin as the others and, therefore, I didn't belong there. I didn't feel worthy to be amongst these women who had achieved so much (as seen through the eyes of one in the throws of anorexia). I felt fat and, once again, I was a failure. At home I was the best, the thinnest, but here it was different. My husband remembers it differently. He remembers walking on to a floor where everyone looked like his emaciated wife. He was horrified that there were so many like me, all of us, one more emaciated than the other, and all striving to be the best. Imagine 20 women of varying ages, together in close quarters, all with severe depression, not one weighing over 90 lbs, all in a state of shell-shock because they really aren't the best at what they had interpreted as being their most valuable and prized personal achievement. Everyone was there to have that achievement taken away from him or her, and not one of us understood why they would want to do such a horrid thing to us. We had all worked so hard to get to where we were and their sole purpose was to destroy this. A common joke among the patients with anorexia, was, 'The best anorexic is the dead anorexic; she wins'. This may be harsh and distasteful, but shows the anorectic mind set. As I gained weight, I found that I was envious of the new people coming into the program. They were thin and I was on the road to getting fat (as I viewed it then). I also found out that this was the same way the residents viewed me as I came in, and the new person felt exactly the same way as I did when I entered the program, the same way everyone felt.

The first two weeks were horrendous. I went in on a long weekend with a skeleton staff on hand. My first meal was lunch. It was put in front of me and I was expected to eat. The first meal was a grace; you didn't have to finish everything. I was horrified at all the food placed in front of me. Prior to my admittance, my entire day's worth of food consumption had consisted of an orange and perhaps a few crackers. The amount of food in front of me seemed unreal, it was like some sort of cruel joke. I sobbed through lunch, managing to eat a few bites through my tears. Supper came all too quickly, as I was still full from lunch, and this time I was expected to eat everything. It was a meat dish (I was a vegetarian), a vegetable, potatoes, a salad, a bun with butter, a yogurt, apple cobbler, juice, an apple and milk (which I didn't drink). All of this was expected to be consumed within 30 minutes. The meals were monitored and the trays checked after the allotted time. Anything left was noted: unused or unfinished butter, a milk carton not empty, an apple not eaten to the core. For two weeks I cried through every meal, as did every new resident. For many weeks I suffered through excruciating stomach pains. There was no help to get through the meals, just a nurse who didn't really want to be there, sitting and staring at all of us. Once we finished, we had to stay in the area for one hour after eating. Anyone needing to use the bathroom was escorted and monitored. You couldn't go to your room. If you forgot your book or journal, then you just sat there, reflecting on the horrid act you just committed against yourself.

There were two psychiatrists assigned to the floor. One lived in the city, and one came in twice a week. The lucky few, who were assigned to the doctor who was on the floor on a daily basis, were the fortunate ones. Each morning they saw him for half an hour. Those of us who had the misfortune to have the other doctor had to wait for his assigned day, not knowing when that day was, as it changed weekly. Any medication problems would have to wait for him. They were reported to the nurse and often changed without even seeing the doctor. On the rare occasion that we actually got to see our doctor, it would be for a maximum of five minutes, at which time only medication was discussed. Suicidal thoughts were considered a personal choice. If you approached a nurse feeling that you couldn't control them, you would be forced to sit in the 'safety chair' in the middle of the hallway outside the nurse's station. Since this was a humiliating experience and did nothing to quell any suicidal thoughts, everyone quickly learned that you didn't approach the nurses at times of trouble. You would receive a lecture on how the thoughts were inappropriate, that it was a way of getting attention, which they didn't have time for, and a threat that any attempt was a first-class ticket to vacate the premises within 24 hours. We all banded together and relied on each other to get through the hard times. We bandaged up each other's self-mutilation wounds, and only approached the nurses when we couldn't handle a suicidal situation or suicide attempt ourselves. Unfortunately, they were the last resort. We did attend classes during the day. These classes brought up issues for everyone; issues which none of us knew how to deal with. That was obvious and inevitable. That's why we were there, that's why we had an eating disorder.

The program was based on weight gain. Upon entry, you were given a goal weight and as you gained weight, you received more privileges. You knew your weight all through the program. If you weren't gaining fast enough, your calorie intake was increased. None of the reasons why you had an eating disorder were addressed. Intense therapy would have made the program much more successful.

Toward the end of my stay at the treatment center, I gave in. I stopped fighting the weight. I just wanted to get out of there. I knew that when I got back home I could lose the weight again; not back to my lowest weight, but to one I was comfortable with, one which I had passed months ago. So I did as I was told, ate what I was told, anything to get out. I did get out. I relapsed one month after discharge. Of course, I got down to the weight I had been comfortable with at the treatment center, but I couldn't stop; I was back in the endless circle of anorexia. Everyone I was in treatment with relapsed as well. Some went on to different treatment centers and some used the tools that they learned and got the help they didn't receive at the center. Some are still in the endless circle of an eating disorder. The experience did provide me with insight into eating disorders and did help bolster my non-existent self-esteem. I was stronger when I finished the program but, unfortunately, without any therapy it didn't help my continuing struggle with my eating disorder.

# Misconceptions: demystifying the eating disorder

There are many misconceptions about eating disorders. In my opinion, the biggest one is that it's a choice that people make in their lives and that one can stop at any time. For me, it wasn't a choice that I consciously made, it just happened. I couldn't stop, even when I wanted to. Perhaps if my eating disorder had been diagnosed earlier, or I had gone into therapy sooner it wouldn't have gone as far as it did. My eating disorder was the way I coped with my life, the way I had control over my life, over the one thing that was truly mine, **my body**. When I speak of praise and envy it could be interpreted as a vanity issue. In order for this to be true, I would have had to like myself. At no time did that happen. No matter how much weight I lost, I still didn't like myself. In fact the opposite was true; I loathed myself even more. The worse I felt about myself, the worse the eating disorder got. It was like an unending circle.

My family and my husband tried various tactics in order to get me to eat. They tried bribery, threats, manipulation and promises. Nothing worked. I wanted it to, but I just couldn't stop. The doctors would try to make me stop by explaining in great detail the consequences to my body. This made no difference. At that point, any consequences were the least of my worries. I couldn't think past the next meal, let alone years or months down the road. Once my eating disorder was fully out of control, I didn't care what damage I was doing. I believed that I wouldn't survive that long anyway. Frankly, I didn't really want to; the pain and torture in my head was so unbearable that the thought of a heart attack or organ failure was comforting. It would put me out of my misery. I honestly believe that the eating disorder was a form of 'passive suicide'.

When I looked in the mirror I saw a horrid fat monster. No one could understand how I could see something different in the mirror than they did. The mirror confirmed for me that I needed to keep dieting, that perhaps at some magic number the fat monster would disappear and I would see what everyone else saw. That never happened. To this day, that hasn't happened. People see what I look like on the outside. What I see is the way I feel about myself on the inside. I see a distorted image of myself turned inside out. I know now about body-image perception distortion, but it's difficult to convince your brain that what your eyes see is not what's really there. For this reason, people don't understand that once you decide to get help, you still fight it. It's because the eating disorder fights harder than you do. It fights with voices in your head.

# The eating disorder voice (EDV)

The voice is the most difficult part of an eating disorder for people to understand. You're afraid to tell anyone, for fear that you'll be labeled psychotic or schizophrenic. The 'EDV' tells you that you're fat, that you are useless, that you are a loser, that if you lose just 5 lbs more, all your problems will go away and you'll be happy. It lies to you, it belittles you, and yet it's your best friend. It's the only thing you can count on. In recovery, you can quiet the voice, talk back to it, but it's still there, fighting to get control back. I've been asked if the voice is of someone I know, my mother, my father, etc. For me it isn't. It's no one I know; it has no shape or form, no identity. I think my 'EDV' is a combination of all the bad things I feel and think about myself put into a voice. It feels like a war going on in your head. It's a living hell. The pain is on the inside, so no one can see. It's hard for people to understand the hell you're going through, because they can't see it. It's not like a broken leg, which people can physically see. It's all on the inside, this horrid war that you fight in your head every day.

# Belief system

My belief system at the time was very simple. Suffering will cleanse the soul. I felt that the more I suffered then, perhaps, somehow it would make me a better person, perhaps even God would forgive me for being such a horrid person. I used examples in my head like Mother Theresa. She lived in squalor and she was happy. She was made a saint! Speaking of saints, they all suffered. They were good human beings. Therefore, if I suffered perhaps I could become a good human being worthy of existence on this earth. My perfectionist thinking came into play here. If I could be perfect and suffer, somehow that would make me into a good person. It all stems from having no self-esteem. If I had any, then I certainly wouldn't have had the belief system that I did.

There were periods of time when I was very proud of myself for what I had accomplished through my eating disorder. The scale kept showing a lower number, therefore I was a success that day. After a long while I realized that no matter what the scale said, I would never be happy. I would never be good enough. The elation would last for several days and then the goal number would have to be lowered. Once that number was reached the same process started again; the pride, the elation and the inevitable spiral down. Once you get to a weight where it's deemed medically critical, panic sets in. Doctors around you start to panic. Part of you can't understand what the big deal is and part of you shares in the panic. You realize that you no longer have any control whatsoever over your eating disorder; in fact, you lost it a long time ago. It now controls you. It controls you through the 'EDV'. At this point, the self-loathing that drove you to a critical weight intensifies. Not only do you hate yourself for all the original reasons, but also now you hate yourself for putting people you love through the heartache of seeing you wither away. Suicidal thoughts fight for time in your head with the EDV. You see no way out. You want to get better, which means gaining weight. At this point this is a sin against oneself. The EDV won't allow you to do this. So you are left in the seemingly never-ending spiral of your eating disorder, alone, unable to express to anyone the torment within you. All the while you put on your 'Happy Mask' and carry on.

# Conclusion

Since no one understood what I was going through and I didn't have the energy or words to describe it all to them, I isolated myself. I stopped seeing friends. I didn't talk to my family. I rarely left the house. I even isolated myself from my husband. I didn't really understand what was happening, so how could I possibly explain it to someone else. It was just easier to be on my own and not inflict my misery on others. Depression also impacted on my self-imposed isolation.

My eating disorder has been with me for over half my life; it feels like it's a part of me. In recovery, it's difficult to separate myself from the eating disorder. I question who I would be without it. It's been my best friend and my worst enemy. Yet, I'm afraid to let go of it. This is the monster I battle to gain control of myself, to find out who I am without my eating disorder. In times of stress it returns like an old friend with promises to take care of me. 'Just give in to me', it says, 'I'll make everything better'. My old friend the EDV. When I no longer have to argue with it, yell at it to stop or to go away, then, at that time, I will truly be free.

# Reference

Stewart M, Brown JB, Weston WW *et al.* (1995) *Patient-Centered Medicine: transforming the clinical method.* Sage Publications, Thousand Oaks, CA.

# 5

# The patient–clinician relationship

The patient–clinician relationship is an essential element in the patient-centered approach to eating disorders and a key ingredient in recovery. The fostering of a collaborative relationship based on trust, a non-judgmental attitude, and a knowledge of the emotional, behavioral and cognitive dynamics of eating disorders is fundamental to the development of 'common ground' during the treatment process. According to Stewart *et al.* (1995), several factors are operative in the development of a therapeutic alliance, including power, caring, healing, self-awareness and issues of transference and countertransference.

The sharing of power and control facilitates a positive and collaborative patient–clinician relationship and promotes the patient's sense of personal efficacy in her own life and her surroundings. The caring attributes demonstrated by the clinician are curative, in that they promote healing by restoring the patient's lost sense of connection to others, well-being and self-control. The clinician's self-awareness is imperative, in that self-knowledge promotes both the personal development of and ability to communicate empathy, genuineness, warmth and respect to the patient.

Transference and countertransference issues are also important considerations in the development of a therapeutic relationship (Stewart *et al.*, 1995). According to Kahn (1997), transference occurs when the patient unconsciously projects or transfers onto the clinician old patterns (attitudes, emotions, expectations) deriving from earlier experiences. Transference may be positive or negative. If positive, it serves to build stronger connections between patient and clinician and provide a corrective emotional experience when interpreted in an empathic and caring way. Within this process, the clinician is not merely a 'blank screen' with no emotions, expressions or attitudes. Rather, patient–clinician interactions are therapeutic to the extent that the clinician functions as a real person who brings his or her humanness to the relationship for the benefit of the patient (Kahn, 1997).

Countertransference encompasses all of the clinician's feelings, attitudes and behavioral reactions toward the patient (Kahn, 1997). It can be obstructive or useful. Obstructive countertransference interferes with the clinician's empathy and clarity in responding to the patient (Kahn, 1997). For example, a clinician who avoids exploring body-image issues with the patient due to his or her own unresolved issues in this area, or who is weight-prejudiced, is engaging in obstructive countertransference. Useful countertransference refers to the clinician's feelings and attitudes which are employed to the patient's advantage (Kahn, 1997). These include genuine, well-timed self-disclosures which foster understanding and rapport and encourage the development of trust and hope in the relationship. The presence of both transference and countertransference underlines the importance of developing self-awareness with regards to unresolved personal issues, values and stressors in clinical training programs and ongoing supervision (Stewart *et al.*, 1995).

This chapter is written from the perspective of three members of the outpatient team, all of whom need to be cognizant of the issues delineated above, both in terms of their relationship with the patient and in terms of their interactions with each other. A psychologist, a physician and a dietitian will describe the patient–clinician relationship in terms of the roles of the clinician, strategies to develop a therapeutic alliance, important attributes of the clinician and unique challenges in treating eating disorders.

# The patient–therapist relationship

## *Kathleen M Berg*

As part of the outpatient team, the individual psychotherapist works in collaboration with all other professionals involved in the patient's care, including the family physician, the dietitian and the family therapist. With the individual's permission, periodic contact with the other members of the team helps to ensure consistency of treatment approach and communication of vital information such as blood test results, proximity to critical weight, suicidal ideation, the impact of a particularly difficult family session, etc. When professionals take responsibility for communicating with each other, it eases some of the frustration and stress experienced by both the sufferer and her family.

# Roles of the therapist

In the patient-centered approach to the treatment of eating disorders, the individual therapist assumes a variety of roles. As a teacher, the therapist imparts expert knowledge about the biology of starvation/bingeing and purging and the psychological (both emotional and cognitive) components of the disorder. This information can empower the patient and enhance her motivation to change. For many individuals, it is a comfort to know that many of their symptoms are a result of being in a state of semi-starvation as opposed to irreversible changes in personality or character flaws. The therapist also teaches the patient about the social context of the disorder and how culture-bound expectations of thinness and perfection have affected her as an individual. Relative to the age of the patient, the therapist discusses the impact of maturational demands such as increased independence, emotional and physical intimacy and coping with changes in body morphology. Skills such as assertiveness and stress management are taught. Finally, the therapist helps the patient to make connections between early experiences and the development of her eating disorder. These experiences may include abuse, parental alcoholism, high performance expectations, loss, childhood obesity, etc.

The individual therapist also functions as a non-coercive coach who bolsters the patient's self-esteem by listening intently to her thoughts and feelings without judgment. The therapist serves as the container of hope for the future and belief in the patient's right and ability to be well and feel good about herself. The effective coach offers encouragement and steadfast support for the patient's right to give birth to her true self (Goodsitt, 1997).

In addition to functioning as a teacher and coach, the individual therapist also serves as a role model for assertion, for emotional labeling and expression, for honoring subjective experience, for recognizing and restructuring self-defeating thoughts and for challenging sociocultural pressures to be thin, passive, silent and selfless. By observing the therapist and interacting with her/him, the patient learns attitudes and behaviors which promote self-esteem, enhance interpersonal skills and help regulate mood.

# Building a therapeutic alliance

In order to maximize the therapeutic alliance, a collaborative approach to individual psychotherapy is advocated. The collaborative approach respects the individual's needs for autonomy and acknowledges her sense of personal ineffectiveness, needs for approval, perfectionism, interpersonal distrust and confusion regarding personal identity. Those with eating disorders are often withdrawn, performance-oriented and fiercely independent. As a result, they may be terrified of becoming close to the therapist and feel panicked about the therapist's expectations. For some patients, there may also be a disavowal of the eating disorder and very low motivation for treatment, As previously stated, this is particularly true of those struggling with anorexia nervosa but may also be found in bulimia nervosa. The therapist needs to be acutely aware of these psychological dynamics, become actively involved and take initial responsibility for establishing rapport. An intuitive appreciation of the 'inner voice' or 'eating disorder voice' and how it torments the patient is crucial in establishing a therapeutic alliance. Whenever possible, the patient should be offered choices and become actively involved in a mutual decision-making process with the therapist.

In the initial phases of therapy, many individuals with eating disorders do not feel entitled to help or they may resist any attempts at intervention. Lecturing and patronizing the patient or treating her like she's inept will likely dissolve any alliance. Comments such as 'Don't you realize what you're doing to your body?', 'You can't fool me, I know you're being manipulative!', and, 'You're just not capable of making logical decisions at this time. You need to relinquish the controls to us', however well-intentioned, are not experienced as helpful by the patient. On the contrary, most patients report that reactions of this sort result in further humiliation, distrust and fears of loss of control. As a result, the patient may actually retreat further into her eating disorder in order to experience feelings of safety and personal control. Similarly, minimization or trivialization of symptoms, as represented by clinician statements such as 'This is just a normal stage of adolescent development', 'You just need to try and eat more', and, 'Just stop eating when you're full', fails to communicate an understanding of the psychological dynamics of the eating disorder and are likely to lead to distrust and alienation. Labeling the individual as 'anorexic' or 'bulimic' also tends to detract from the therapeutic alliance. Language has subtle powers. The patient needs to be viewed as a whole and unique person who has an eating disorder rather than a case of anorexia nervosa versus bulimia nervosa.

A therapist who focuses exclusively on food and weight issues and makes weight gain or cessation of bingeing and purging the sole aim of therapy is often viewed by patients as being indifferent to her inner suffering, especially as time goes on. This reality often eludes the therapist, particularly when the patient is successful at engaging her or him in endless discussions about the details of her eating behavior or arguments about the true gravity of her disorder. Failure to address the inner world of the patient can result in withdrawal, anger and even contempt as expressed by a young adolescent recently discharged from a hospital program and currently being seen as an outpatient: 'They're all happy because I weigh what they want me to and they think I'm better. They didn't care. They thought they knew me but they didn't. They didn't know how hard it is and nobody really talked to me. Fine! Now that I'm out of there, I'm just going to lose it all again and they can't do anything about it!' The underlying plea to the current therapist is: 'Please be compassionate and see my pain. Please know that I'm hurting on the inside even when I act like everything is fine. Please understand that I really am trying, there are forces operating inside me that confuse and frighten me'.

There are essential personal characteristics required of the therapist who chooses to engage in the treatment of eating disorders. As previously stated, anorexia nervosa and bulimia nervosa are complex, challenging problems. Treatment tends to be long-term, and relapses are common. In a patient-centered approach to treatment, the following qualities and the ability to communicate them to the patient effectively are viewed as important contributors to the development of an therapeutic alliance:

- empathic understanding
- non-judgmental acceptance
- patience, optimism and emotional fortitude. Impatience, pessimism and anxiety on the part of the therapist results in feelings of defeat and hopelessness for the patient. The therapist needs to remain calm but take the patient seriously
- warmth and compassion and an ability to instill trust and create a safe place for the sufferer
- flexibility and a willingness to negotiate
- alertness and clarity; the therapist must stay tuned into signs of relapse and the patient's reactions to the therapist and to the treatment progress
- self-awareness; self-knowledge regarding personal issues and values impacts the clinician's consciousness of and ability to work through issues of transference and countertransference as defined in the introduction to this chapter
- humility; the treatment of eating disorders is a humbling experience; we have much to learn from each patient about the effectiveness and ineffectiveness of alternative treatments.

According to Strober (1997), both expert knowledge and the specified qualities of the therapist are essential ingredients to the establishment of a therapeutic bond and eventual success in treatment. 'If the therapist is lacking in these qualities or is of rigid bearing, the initial encounter will be deprived of vital elements ... treatment of this illness is slippery and time-consuming and the stakes are high. Not all therapists are prepared to begin such undertakings and some will be poorly suited for work with this population.'

# Unique challenges in the therapeutic relationships

Denial and distortion, imposed treatment and treatment refusal, initial views of the therapist as the 'enemy', and issues related to body image are common challenges in the individual treatment of anorexia nervosa and bulimia nervosa.

Denial and distortion from the patient's point of view were discussed in Chapter 3. The challenge for the therapist is to acknowledge the patient's feelings and beliefs without judgment while continuing to offer her a new perspective, by agreeing to disagree, by employing gentle, tentative confrontations and by openly anticipating and discussing emotional reactions including any disavowal of the disorder. Close collaboration with the patient on the establishment of therapy goals and treatment plans maximizes engagement in the process and minimizes fear and distrust.

Whenever possible, therapists should be patient with initial treatment refusal and avoid imposed interventions. The negative emotional consequences of using force can be profound and result in an aversion to any form of treatment. In individual psychotherapy, the door to engagement in the therapeutic process may not be the eating disorder *per se* but the patient's unhappiness, stress or frustrations with family/peer relationships. One can build up an alliance through these channels first.

Goldner *et al.* (1997) have written an excellent discussion on the clinical, ethical and legal considerations involved in treatment refusal. While many of their comments relate specifically to inpatient treatment programs, their recommendations are valuable considerations for application to individual psychotherapy on an outpatient basis. It is advisable to introduce the possibility of hospitalization or entry into a treatment program early in therapy. In addition, therapists should not assume that initial refusals are final. Tact, compassion, information and growing trust in the therapist often result in relief in having others make the decisions. This gives the patient 'permission' to eat and in her eyes diminishes the guilt, shame and fear she experiences in nourishing herself. The following recommendations are among those offered by Goldner *et al.* (1997):

- seek to engage in a sincere and voluntary alliance
- identify the reasons for refusal
- provide careful explanations of treatment recommendations
- be prepared for negotiations
- promote autonomy
- weigh the risks vs benefits of imposed treatment
- avoid battles and scare tactics
- convey a balance of control vs non-control (a firm communication of necessary constraints within a flexible framework)
- ensure that treatment methods are not inherently punitive
- involve the family where appropriate
- conceptualize refusal/resistance as an evolutionary process wherein patients can change their minds over time.

A related challenge is presented to the therapist when the patient views him or her as the 'enemy' who is trying to make her 'fat', taking away her 'biggest accomplishment', robbing her of the right to control her own body or trying to make her 'submit'. The patient may be very critical and harbor mistrust of all health professionals. It takes a great deal of fortitude, energy and unfailing empathy to avoid power struggles with the patient and resist personalizing accusations. When the eating disorder is severe, it can be heart-breaking to observe the suffering which patients and their families endure. The lack of adequate inpatient treatment programs, support groups and/or family physicians who are knowledgeable about and sympathetic to the struggles of patients with eating disorders can be an added burden for the individual psychotherapist. On the other hand, it is tremendously rewarding to participate in a process which involves the emotional, physical, relational and spiritual healing of someone and wrestle the control away from an eating disorder to put it back where it belongs, with the individual.

Another unique challenge in the patient/therapist relationship concerns issues related to body image. These factors are likely to surface more with female therapists than with males who work in this area. Some patients may scrutinize the therapist's body and feel a competitive edge if she perceives herself to be thinner than the therapist. Conversely, the clinician whose body reflects the sociocultural ideals of thin, fit and perfectly shaped may be a threat to some patients. The patient's own weight prejudice may lead her to undermine the therapist's competence, particularly if she views the therapist as overweight. As a result, clinicians working with individuals who struggle with anorexia nervosa or bulimia nervosa need to be aware of and have worked through their personal issues around body image including weight prejudice. Furthermore, the therapist needs to be willing to openly respond to these issues when they arise over the course of treatment.

# Role of the physician

*James A McSherry*

The relationship between patients and physicians is the foundation stone of any mutually satisfactory clinical interaction. Without a human connection, patients and physicians are likely to be left feeling that something important has been missed. The patient brings an illness to the physician's office, the physician seeks to diagnose a disease. The patient's complaints are one thing, but his or her needs, as defined by the physician, may be something else entirely. The physician's medical advice may be scrupulously correct, but the patient's needs may go unrecognized when medical interactions are disease-focused or doctor-centered (Mishler, 1984). Patient-centered medicine (Stewart *et al.*, 1995) provides a means of accommodating the physician's technical approach and the patient's human needs for understanding.

The patient's ideas, expectations and feelings about an illness, together with its effect on function, the four dimensions of the illness experience, are important determinants of patient satisfaction with any clinical encounter. They are many times more powerful when those encounters are between physicians and patients with eating disorders.

# Strategies to develop therapeutic alliance

Eating disorders tend to evolve over time and few affected persons consistently portray a single uniform clinical presentation. Instead, most patients with eating disorders display a variety of behaviors of different degrees of severity along a continuum that includes the entities diagnosable as anorexia nervosa and bulimia nervosa. The physician may be concerned about malnutrition at one visit when food restriction may be the dominant characteristic, or about electrolyte imbalance at another when reports of frequent and severe purging suggest an electrolyte imbalance. These are legitimate and important issues for the knowledgeable and competent physician, but they may not be great concerns for patients operating from different attitudes and beliefs. The ability to maintain a low-calorie diet may actually be a source of satisfaction to the patient whose life is dominated by fear of fatness, and purging may be seen as a legitimate approach to avoid weight gain in a patient who has eating binges.

Management strategies must be flexible and allow modifications that accommodate changes in the patient's agenda. The patient's focus at one visit might be management of specific eating-disorder symptoms, while at another it may be mood disturbance or problems with personal relationships. The physician's perpetual concern in such a situation is to relate the patient's ideas, expectations and feelings to the effect of the illness on function, and to find the common ground that allows patient and physician to grow together in their understanding of how the patient's unique experience of the illness shapes her response to the physician's advice.

A trusting therapeutic relationship is fundamental to the whole process of helping affected persons accept their eating disorders, engage in treatment and move to recovery. Without the trusting relationship, professional helpers are viewed as just wanting to make their patients fat. After all, in anorexia nervosa we seek to have our patients gain weight, the very focus of their anxiety, and in bulimia nervosa to stop the maladaptive behavior that kept them from getting fat in the first place.

# Important attributes of the physician

Persons affected by eating disorders value physicians who are optimistic in outlook, realistic in expectation, non-judgemental in attitude, patient with their progress, knowledgeable about their condition and sensitive to their fears. A physician's willingness to work along with patients is highly prized, as is recognition and acceptance that not all progress will be forward and absolute compliance always unlikely.

### Case study: the story of Joanne

Joanne was a 23-year-old graduate student who consulted a physician about her acne. It was the first time she had seen this particular physician although her troubles with acne had gone on for a number of years. As she explained during the interview, her acne had begun to be a nuisance about five years earlier. She had consulted her family physician at first and she had prescribed various topical agents and a series of antibiotics before referring her to a dermatologist when the acne failed to respond. The dermatologist recommended a four-month course of Accutane, a powerful oral medication that cleared up her acne for at least a year and a half. The purpose of her visit on this occasion was to ask for another course of Accutane, since her acne had broken out again and seemed to be heading in the same florid direction as before the first treatment.

The physician acknowledged the severity of Joanne's acne and stated that he had no objection to prescribing another course of Accutane if necessary. However, to Joanne's surprise, he began to ask her about her menstrual cycle. He was particularly interested in her age at menarche (when her periods first began), the date of her last menstrual period, the frequency of her periods and the interval between them. He explained that severe acne was sometimes the first indication of a hormone imbalance in young women and irregular periods could be another sign of the same thing. Joanne was intrigued by this suggestion as her periods had in fact been irregular over the previous six months and it was the first time anyone had brought the subject up. She had never thought to ask a physician about her menstrual cycle as she hadn't thought it important since she wasn't sexually active. She was particularly interested when the physician commented that other signs of the hormonal imbalance included a tendency to gain weight despite diet and exercise. She readily agreed to have some blood taken for laboratory tests and arranged another appointment a week later.

Her next appointment was a bit of a shock for her. The physician told her that his suspicions of a hormonal imbalance were confirmed by the finding that her serum free testosterone was above normal, although her total serum testosterone was normal. The physician explained that women produce a small amount of testosterone, a male hormone, just as men produce a small amount of estrogen, a female hormone. Her own testosterone was present in her body in two forms, one bound to serum proteins and one that circulated free in an unbound form. The unbound form is biologically active and even small increases in the free testosterone level could produce clinically significant effects such as acne, excessive bodily hair, menstrual disturbance and weight gain. The whole condition was probably the result of a minor metabolic error at the level of her ovaries. Treatment of the condition was not difficult at this stage in her life.

Joanne was shocked when the physician went on to say that there had been another abnormal blood test ... her serum potassium was low. The physician told her that low potassium levels could be the result of vomiting, or diarrhea and asked her if she had suffered a tummy upset before her first visit, or if she was taking medication, a diuretic, for example, that might explain this finding. Joanne responded by denying diuretic use. The physician went on to say that low potassium levels in young women were sometimes an indication of repeated vomiting or laxative abuse as a weight-control measure. Joanne didn't answer for a few moments and then admitted that she had been very frustrated by her inability to control her weight over the last year, had attempted to restrict her calorie intake, but found herself having periodic eating binges that led to self-induced vomiting after eating binges when her weight gain worsened. A friend had been dieting successfully at the same time, and this had just added to her frustration.

After taking a detailed history of her eating behavior, the physician concluded that Joanne was struggling with bulimia nervosa in addition to her hormone imbalance, a condition he called 'an androgen-excess syndrome.' Joanne was very relieved that her weight-control problem was now out in the open as it had been a serious concern for her, one that she had not felt able to confide in to anyone, not even her closest friends. She was particularly relieved to hear that both conditions were related and that treatment of the androgen-excess syndrome would help bring her weight under control.

Some further investigations were organized and Joanne agreed to start taking an oral contraceptive as a means of controlling the hormonal imbalance. Additionally, she readily agreed to a series of appointments for counseling regarding the eating disorder, as she had been favorably impressed by the physician's knowledge, courteous approach and willingness to explain things as they went along, together with the direct non-judgmental style that had led her to confide in him in the first place.

# Unique challenges for the physician

Eating disorders rarely respond to short-term interventions and it is often diffi-cult for the physician to see progress. Frustration, and perhaps guilt, may color the physician's attitude to the patient and activate countertransference. The wise physician is sufficiently professional, self-aware and insightful to recognize this as a major issue. In the author's experience as a physician and teacher, case discussions with colleagues in a collaborative multidisciplinary team are often helpful in these situations and obtaining a formal consultation from a know-ledgeable colleague may provide useful suggestions that allow physician and patient to move beyond problematic issues.

# The patient–dietitian relationship

*Nancy E Strange*

# Role of the dietitian

The role of the dietitian as a member of the treatment team involves not only nutritional assessment and nutrition education, but also interpretation of disordered eating behaviors, communication with other team members and provision of ongoing support for the patient in the recovery process. The recov-ery process for the person suffering from an eating disorder involves:

- long-term care
- a significant relationship, that in and of itself is a key part of the recovery process
- a treatment plan that is highly individualized and evolves over time (Reiff and Lampton Reiff, 1992).

# Building a therapeutic relationship

First and foremost, the dietitian must work on establishing an atmosphere that is non-threatening to the patient. It is not uncommon for a person suffering from an eating disorder to have difficulties with persons in positions of author-ity. This may be due to previous experiences, either before or during the course of her eating disorder. She may arrive with preconceived ideas of being judged and berated for her eating behaviors, particularly if she has had this experience in the past. It is therefore very useful to ask the patient at the first visit what her expectations are and what she hopes to obtain from nutrition therapy. The responses received will vary widely among individuals. If the dietitian is empathetic and non-judgmental in listening to the patient's needs at this time, that will help set the stage for a positive working relationship. It will then be up to the dietitian to tailor a nutrition treatment plan to meet those expectations. In this way the dietitian and the patient will be collaborating to meet the needs of the individual patient. In order to establish a successful therapeutic relationship, it is critical that the patient be aware that she can trust the dietitian. This trust must cover many areas. She needs to feel confident in her trust that the dietitian will give her accurate information, and not try to 'trick' her into eating foods she has fears of by making false claims about them. She needs to know that she can trust the dietitian not to 'make her fat' by any specific recommendations or meal plans that she might provide. That trust must also extend to keeping confidences as requested, unless they are related to activities which could prove dangerous to her well-being.

It is important to bear in mind that it may take several sessions with an individual suffering from an eating disorder, in order to build a solid therapeutic alliance. If the patient has had previous negative experiences with healthcare professionals, she will be slow to trust. This process of establishing a strong therapeutic relationship requires patience, but is well worth waiting for. Working with a patient with an eating disorder may well be overall one of the most challenging but consequently also one of the most rewarding experiences a dietitian may have.

# Attributes patients look for in a dietitian

There are certain expectations that the person suffering from an eating disorder will have of the dietitian, and if the dietitian cannot fulfill these requirements, it will be very difficult for her or him to assist the patient in her recovery. Some of these expectations will be related to specific abilities and some will actually be personal attributes or qualities.

Personal attributes a person suffering from an eating disorder may look for in a dietitian include the following:

- **calm and patient:** The dietitian must allow the patient to move forward at her own pace, and be comfortable with slow improvement; if she is displaying signs of impatience with the patient's slow rate of improvement, this will add to the patient's stress in the recovery process

- **supportive:** The patient is looking for a dietitian with a positive attitude, and an ability to provide strength and support at particularly difficult times
- **flexible:** It is often necessary to revise plans and treatment programs as time goes by and situations change, and it is important for the dietitian to be able to do that without regarding the patient as 'manipulative'
- **role model regarding healthy eating style and positive body image:** It is helpful if the patient actually 'sees' the dietitian eating a normal meal, rather than just talking about it; also the dietitian must have worked through any issues she or he has regarding body image, so that she or he reflects a positive body image for her/himself, regardless of actual body build
- **good level of comfort in working with an individual with an eating disorder:** A dietitian may have an excellent level of nutrition knowledge and plenty of information regarding eating disorders, obtained from literature; but if he or she is not comfortable with all of the 'baggage' that a patient with an eating disorder brings, and has difficulty with all the feelings involved, she or he will not likely be successful in helping in the recovery process
- **empathetic:** The dietitian will be much more useful to the patient if able to imaginatively enter into the patient's feelings about her situation
- **compassion:** One must have the heart to work with these clients as many have been abused, abandoned or neglected, and they are wounded and often very angry; all the knowledge in the world cannot replace compassion (Hahn, 1998).

Let us now consider the professional qualities that a person suffering from an eating disorder looks for in a dietitian.

- **Expertise in nutritional care.** The patient has a right to expect that a qualified, registered dietitian will bring to this relationship expert nutrition knowledge to use in the processes of nutritional assessment and nutrition therapy.
- **Excellent level of knowledge of eating disorders.** In order to be of value to the patient in the recovery process, the dietitian must also have extensive cognizance of eating disorders and the effects they have on a sufferer's life.
- **Ability to collaborate with, rather than control, the patient.** Collaboration truly is the key to a successful recovery. If the patient does not have 'ownership' of her recovery plan, she will not likely be empowered to fully participate.
- **Ability to listen.** Dietitians are trained to talk and to teach, but not usually how to listen. Often the most important thing the dietitian does in the first few session is to really listen to the patient, and get a sense of how she feels and what her experiences have been.
- **Realistic expectations.** The dietitian must realize that recovery from an eating disorder is usually a very long and difficult process. It is very different

from dealing with a patient who just needs education and a plan to promote weight gain. One must be forever cognizant of the intense emotions regarding eating experienced by a person suffering from an eating disorder.

- **Ability to 'jump-start' the patient when she gets 'stuck'.** It is typical for a person recovering from an eating disorder to go a distance down the road to recovery, and then 'park' for a while in order to achieve a level of comfort with the particular stage she is at. This is normal and very acceptable. However, if she 'parks' for too long, she runs the risk of getting stuck at this point in her recovery. She needs a dietitian who can gently confront her on this issue and help her to 'start her engine' again.

- **Optimism regarding recovery.** At all times it is necessary for the dietitian to maintain an optimistic outlook regarding the patient's recovery. If the patient perceives that any member of the treatment team regards her as hopeless, she will have a great deal of difficulty in putting her best efforts into her recovery. Sandra demonstrated this fact very well. On her first visit to the dietitian's office she stated that every dietitian and every psychiatrist she had ever seen had give up on her and considered her 'hopeless', and that this dietitian probably would too. It was clear she was testing the dietitian. She was told that day that this dietitian would never give up on her. She needed this reassurance. Sandra has now maintained a healthy body weight for over a year. She has returned to school and is preparing for a career. She attributes this success to the fact that she finally found a dietitian and a psychiatrist who believed in her, were optimistic about her ability to recover and never gave up on her.

When working with a patient with an eating disorder, the dietitian must be aware of countertransference issues. This involves the arousal of the dietitian's own feelings through identification with the patient's experiences or problems. An example of this might be a dietitian who had experienced weight-control problems in her own adolescence, and suffered with low self-esteem during that struggle. If she still carries those emotional scars, even though the weight is no longer a problem, she may have a great deal of difficulty in being truly objective in her dealings with the patient. It is critical that the dietitian resolve any issues of her own, in order not to actually interfere with the recovery of the patient.

# Conclusion

Clearly there are many common themes to the patient–clinician relationship, whether viewed from the perspective of the therapist, the physician or the dietitian. The healing process is a long one and a comfortable relationship where power and control are truly shared is absolutely essential.

The patient needs to feel confident not only in the knowledge and expertise of the clinicians she is working with, but also in their personal and professional attributes. She needs to know that she is working with non-judgmental individuals in whom she can trust. A positive atmosphere where the patient and clinician can collaborate to form goals and plans for recovery helps to foster the healing process.

Team collaboration is also an important aspect in this process. In order to provide the best care and support for the patient, the clinicians must communicate with each other to increase their awareness of all important issues. All communication should be done with the patient's permission.

A good team of clinicians working together with the patient will foster a strong alliance that will not only assist the patient along the road to recovery, but also make the road less 'rocky'.

# References

Goldner EM, Birmingham CL and Smye V (1997) Addressing treatment refusal in anorexia nervosa: clinical, ethical and legal considerations. In: DM Garner and PE Garfinkel (eds) *Handbook of Treatment for Eating Disorders*. Guilford Press, New York.

Goodsitt A (1997) Eating disorders: a self-psychological perspective. In: DM Garner and PE Garfinkel (eds) *Handbook of Treatment for Eating Disorders*. Guilford Press, New York.

Hahn NI (1998) When food becomes a cry for help. *J Am Diet Assoc.* **98**(4): 395–8.

Kahn M (1997) *Between Therapist and Client: the new relationship*. WH Freeman & Co, New York.

Mishler EG (1984) *Discourse of Medicine: dialectics of medical interviews*. Ablex, Norwood, NJ.

Reiff DW and Lampson Reiff KK (1992) The role of the nutrition therapist. In: *Eating Disorders, Nutrition Therapy in the Recovery Process*. Aspen Publishers, Inc, Gathersburg, MD.

Stewart M, Brown JB, Weston WW *et al.* (1995) *Patient-Centered Medicine: transforming the clinical method*. Sage Publications, Thousand Oaks, CA.

Strober M (1997) Consultation and therapeutic engagement in severe anorexia nervosa. In: DM Garner and PE Garfinkel (eds) *Handbook of Treatment for Eating Disorders*. Guilford Press, New York.

# 6

# Management and finding common ground

A patient-centered approach to the management of eating disorders is a collaborative endeavor based on mutual understanding and agreement on identification and prioritizing of patient concerns, treatment goals and the changing roles of the clinician and the patient in the recovery process. This approach is an ongoing interactive process which fosters the development of common ground and incorporates the patient's feelings, ideas, function and expectations, as described in Chapter 3, in treatment planning (Stewart *et al.*, 1995).

This chapter takes an in-depth look at the work of four key clinicians who deal with eating-disordered patients and their families. Perspectives are offered from psychology, family therapy, nutrition and family medicine. In the patient-centered approach, open communication among these members of the outpatient team is also important. Information sharing and collaborative decision-making within the team regarding treatment goals, options for therapeutic intervention and patient progress further develops common ground. Finally, there is a section on the experience of the patient who, in the end, is the final arbitrator of what is helpful and what is not helpful.

We begin with a section on individual and group therapy, which explores the many options available to the eating-disordered patient in the spectrum of psychological interventions for eating disorders. The importance of responding to the unique experience of each patient is emphasized. The development of common ground is encouraged through collaboration between the patient and the therapist.

Family therapy interventions are reviewed in the following section, as well as the importance of the family therapist being clinically experienced with eating-disordered families. It is important that the correct balance between the family's expectations of treatment and the patients' views of what the role of the family in the recovery process should be is explored.

Nutritional management is then reviewed in detail, with the goal of normalizing eating habits and reviewing barriers to normal eating. The emphasis is on personal health and well-being rather than weight.

An overview of management from the family physician's perspective is provided which looks first at medical complications that arise in the management of patients with eating disorders. A brief review of the major medications that are routinely prescribed is included.

Lastly, the patient speaks about her experience of treatment and the effect of the various aspects of her care in the recovery process. It is an essential 'corrective voice' that helps clinicians redesign their interventions towards the best possible outcome for the individual patient.

# Individual psychotherapy and group therapy

*Kathleen M Berg*

Individual or one-on-one psychotherapy may be offered by a psychologist, psychiatrist, social worker or other trained professional. In general, individual psychotherapy involves the structured use of the professional relationship to enable the person to discover, explore and express aspects of herself in order to bring about healthy patterns of behavior and manage subjective distress. Therefore, rather than using concrete interventions such as medication and surgical procedures, individual psychotherapists rely on themselves and their relationship with the patient as the primary agent of treatment and therapeutic change. This fundamental premise cuts across all theoretical models. The models most relevant to the treatment of eating disorders include interpersonal psychotherapy, psychodynamic approaches, cognitive-behavioral therapy and the feminist approach to therapy. While these approaches differ in terms of theoretical orientation and specific intervention strategies, the general treatment goals are the same:

- weight restoration and reversal of physical, emotional and behavioral symptoms of starvation
- improvement in eating behavior (elimination of self-starvation, binge eating, purging)
- increased self-esteem
- improvement in social functioning.

# Interpersonal psychotherapy

Interpersonal psychotherapy (Fairburn, 1997) is a comparatively short-term form of therapy designed to help patients identify and modify current interpersonal difficulties. Originally formulated for the short-term treatment of depression, interpersonal psychotherapy has received moderate empirical support for the treatment of bulimia nervosa. Unlike cognitive-behavioral therapy, this approach is non-directive and does not focus directly on eating problems or underlying attitudes about weight and shape.

Interpersonal psychotherapy for eating disorders is divided into three stages (Fairburn, 1997). In the first stage, the therapist seeks to identify the patient's interpersonal problems that contributed to the development and maintenance of the eating disorder. Interpersonal difficulties are assessed according to four standard 'problem areas'. These include:

- the grief process and unresolved feelings of guilt, anger and sadness surrounding the loss
- interpersonal role disputes and unresolved conflicts
- problems with role transitions and struggles in establishing independence
- interpersonal deficits as exemplified by social isolation and long-term difficulties in establishing intimate relationships.

The second stage involves the establishment of a therapeutic contract for working on the identified interpersonal problems. Stage three addresses termination issues, including strategies for maintaining treatment progress when regular sessions have ended and minimizing the risk of relapse.

# Psychodynamic psychotherapy

Psychodynamic psychotherapies tend to be long-term and are based on the assumption that eating disorders are actually symptoms of underlying internal conflicts. Rather than focus directly on the disordered eating behaviors and dysfunctional thoughts, these approaches are concerned with psychosocial, psychosexual and maturational conflicts. Self-psychologists (Goodsitt, 1997), for example, emphasize parental failures to respond appropriately to a child's needs for validation, acceptance, safety and support. These failures lead to deficits in abilities to maintain self-esteem, identify and express needs and cope with shifts in moods. As a result, the individual is vulnerable to developing an eating disorder. Crisp (1997) conceptualizes anorexia nervosa as a 'flight from growth' and focuses on maturational problems at puberty. These problems result in extreme avoidance of normal adult body weight and shape and associated pressures towards dealing with sexuality and intimacy issues. The fear of confronting adulthood is displaced (transferred) onto food. Psychotherapy is aimed at promoting self-support, self-esteem and social skills and resolving fears of growing up. During this process, the therapist explains and interprets the disordered eating as a manifestation of deeper problems and functions as a coach for the development of communication skills.

# Cognitive-behavioral therapy

Cognitive-behavioral therapy has received considerable empirical support as the treatment of choice for bulimia nervosa and has recently been adapted for the treatment of anorexia nervosa (Garner *et al.*, 1997). In the cognitive-behavioral approach advocated by Garner *et al.* (1997), therapy operates along two intersecting 'tracks'. The first track concentrates on behaviors aimed at weight control, including severe dieting, binge eating, purging and excessive exercise. The second track pertains to psychological themes such as perfectionism, need for approval, emotional expression, self-concept, personal control, impulse regulation, family conflicts and interpersonal functioning. Both tracks are characterized by dysfunctional thoughts, irrational beliefs and reasoning errors. During the initial phases of treatment, more emphasis is placed on track one. The focus here is on conscious experience in the 'here-and-now'. Patients are encouraged to follow behavioral assignments, such as keeping food charts and monitoring thoughts, moods and exercise outside the session. Despite initial resistance from some individuals, self-monitoring can be a very effective tool in regaining control over eating. Strategies are taught which serve to interrupt the binge/purge cycle and new eating patterns are prescribed (i.e. 'mechanical eating' to take away the anxiety of making decisions around food, spacing food intake to minimize cravings, increasing the range of foods consumed). As progress is made in the areas of eating behavior and weight, the treatment emphasis gradually shifts to track two issues.

Throughout the course of therapy, the patient is taught to identify dysfunctional thoughts and reasoning errors which influence her perceptions, emotions and behaviors and which serve to further entrench her in the eating disorder. Examples of dysfunctional thoughts or cognitive distortions were presented in Chapter 2. In the initial phases of treatment, attention is more often focussed on irrational ideas about food and weight. Over time, increased attention is paid to the track two issues of low self-esteem, emotional awareness/expression and relationships. Cognitive restructuring is a treatment strategy which teaches the patient to examine and modify dysfunctional thinking. Garner *et al.* (1997) have identified several steps in the development of cognitive restructuring skills:

- monitoring thoughts and increasing awareness of thought patterns
- identifying and articulating dysfunctional beliefs or thoughts
- examining evidence for and against the validity and utility of each dysfunctional belief

- drawing a reasonable conclusion based on this evidence
- experimenting with behavioral changes that are consistent with this conclusion
- developing believable disputing or challenging thoughts and interpretations more based in reality
- gradually modifying underlying assumptions which generate the dysfunctional thoughts and beliefs: for example, many of those with eating disorders have a basic underlying belief that they are not worthwhile, and the assumption that one has no personal worth colors one's perceptions in many areas and results in negative, self-defeating thoughts such as: 'I do not deserve to eat today' or 'I can't be a very good person if I am not the smartest in the class', or 'I have to work all the time to make up for being such a failure'.

In the final phase of treatment, the cognitive-behavioral therapist prepares the patient for termination and teaches specific strategies to reduce the likelihood of relapse. Relapse prevention includes a review of warning signs, identification of individual areas of vulnerability (i.e. times of major life transitions, personal loss, pregnancy, work or school stress, difficult relationships) and summarization of cognitive and behavioral coping strategies which have proved effective for this particular individual.

# The feminist approach

The feminist approach to individual psychotherapy (Brown, 1993; Hutchinson, 1994) underlines the importance of acknowledging the social and political context within which eating disorders develop. It may be viewed as a philosophy or orientation challenging traditional approaches that focus solely on the pathology of anorexia nervosa and bulimia nervosa, make assumptions based on male-based models of psychological development and fail to incorporate research findings based on the psychology of women. The feminist therapist recognizes that women's problem-solving process is relational and founded on emotions and connections with others as well as logic and rationality. An understanding of the impact of differential power and gender-role stereotyping on the roles which women carry in this culture, the biology of the female lifecycle and women's sexuality are all important in the feminist approach. Therapists focus on the empowerment of women and challenge treatment programs that control and define women's needs and choices for them. Brown (1993), for example, feels that many inpatient and outpatient programs are overfocused on changing the symptoms (dieting, bingeing, purging) without addressing underlying abuse, self-esteem and personal identity issues. Treatment programs which punish, control and manage women's behavior are viewed as fuelling power struggles between the therapist and the individual who is desperately seeking control over her body and her own life. According to Brown (1993), this struggle is then reframed as the woman's problem: she is viewed as unco-operative, manipulative and sick. The feminist approach calls for non-coercive and non-violating treatment strategies.

Feminist therapists acknowledge that in Western society today, girls and women are speaking with their bodies and this voice must be heard, both by the therapist and by the woman herself. Therapy is focused on rebuilding self-esteem, fostering self-direction and validating individual needs and feelings. Victimization (sexual abuse, physical/emotional abuse, sexual harassment, sexism, etc.), role conflicts, and identity confusion are common themes. The feminist therapist functions as a partner and facilitator who collaborates with the individual and offers her knowledge, skills and compassion. The therapist needs to be aware of her own body image issues and weight prejudices and how these impact on the therapeutic relationship. Finally, this approach to psychotherapy recognizes and respects the diversity of women's experience in terms of age, marital status, race, sexual orientation and cultural background. These unique backgrounds affect body image, eating behavior, sex roles and interpersonal relationships. Feminist therapy seeks to honor these differences by individualizing treatments to meet girls' and women's unique needs.

# A patient-centered, multimodal approach to individual psychotherapy

In-keeping with the view that anorexia nervosa and bulimia nervosa are multi-dimensional in nature, an integrated, multimodal approach to individual psychotherapy is advocated. This treatment approach capitalizes on the strengths of the major theoretical models and is individually tailored to meet the unique needs of the individual. The basic philosophy of the feminist approach is advocated because it is patient-centered and recognizes the unique experience of each patient. Furthermore, the approach is collaborative, includes the patient in the decision-making process and addresses the varied sociocultural issues, individual predispositions, interpersonal factors and traumatic experiences which contribute to the development and maintenance of anorexia nervosa and bulimia nervosa.

Cognition distortions are a central feature of eating disorders. These distortions are related to both food and weight issues and deeper issues of identity, self-esteem, body image and interpersonal difficulties. Failure to address self-defeating thought patterns can further entrench the individual in the disorder and heighten chances of relapse. One strength of the cognitive-behavioral approach lies in its direct interventions with both the thought processes and the eating behaviors. It is collaborative and empowers the patient by teaching her self-enhancing and adaptive skills.

Many cognitive-behavioral therapists advocate the use of psychoeducational materials as an adjunct to individual therapy. According to Garner (1997), the psychoeducation component of treatment fosters a collaborative relationship by conveying the message that the responsibility for change rests with the patient. This stance is aimed at reducing defensiveness and enhancing motivation. Common psychoeducational issues include the following:

- the myths of dieting
- the effects of starvation and chaotic eating on emotions, behavior, cognitions and the physical body
- strategies aimed at restoring weight and regular eating patterns: these include skills to manage binge eating and purging and strategies for the development of 'conscious eating'
- education regarding the sociocultural context of the eating disorder and the impact of the media on body image and self-esteem.

In addition, most patients benefit greatly from specific skills training in the areas of stress management and assertion. These skills can replace self-starvation and bingeing/purging as coping methods in dealing with emotional distress and interpersonal problems.

Finally, the cognitive-behavioral approach to individual psychotherapy explicitly teaches the patient to watch for signs of relapse and encourages 'booster sessions' in follow-up and aftercare. Box 6.1 provides a list of warning signs of possible relapse in anorexia nervosa and bulimia nervosa. Therapists need to explain warning signs in concrete, understandable terms. With the permission of the individual, inclusion of significant others can be helpful in the early recognition of signs of relapse.

The multimodal approach also advocates the application of an insight-oriented component (i.e. interpersonal psychotherapy, psychodynamic therapy, self-psychology) to explore the meaning and impact of previous experiences (parental messages, abuse, loss, inadequate nurturing) on the intrapsychic (self-concept, self-esteem, identity, sexuality) world of the patient.

Finally, a multidimensional approach to the treatment of eating disorders makes use of experiential approaches such as art therapy, journal writing, creative visualization and movement therapy when appropriate. The experiential component may be offered by the individual therapist or someone who specializes in the particular area. In the author's experience, these approaches are effective in promoting emotional expression and in accessing spirituality and creative aspects of the self. Body-oriented approaches such as movement (dance, yoga, tai chi, therapeutic massage, and deep muscle relaxation) can help the individual

**Box 6.1:** *Warning signs of relapse with an eating disorder*

- An increase in obsessive thinking about food, weight or shape
- Recognizing increased self-defeating thought patterns, e.g. all-or-nothing thinking
- Experiencing urges to diet - skipping meals, forgetting to eat, counting calories or fat grams, cutting back on portions
- Experiencing urges to binge-eat
- Experiencing urges to vomit or abuse laxatives
- Believing that one can purge 'just once'
- Beginning to think/feel obsessively about exercise in order to compensate for food intake
- Ignoring pain and/or exhaustion when exercising
- Becoming dependent on weight or size to determine success or happiness
- Believing one is fat even when others view one as thin
- Increased social isolation
- Fantasizing about perfection as a way to feel better, e.g. imagining the perfect body, the perfect mark at school, the perfect relationship, etc.
- Constantly scrutinizing one's body in the mirror or dread of seeing one's body
- Drinking excessive amounts of water, coffee or diet pop to trick oneself into believing one has maintained weight or is not hungry
- Using food consumption or dieting to 'solve' problems with stress, anxiety, anger, conflict
- Providing self or others with inaccurate reports (exaggerated or minimized) about symptoms – eating behavior, troublesome thoughts or feelings
- Feeling anxious about decisions around food, eating the same foods all the time, choosing only low-calorie/low-fat foods, chaotic eating patterns, rapid, unconscious eating
- Feeling out of control
- Hiding emotions (anxiety, depression, anger, guilt) from others including the therapist
- Inability to tolerate the feeling of food in one's stomach; feeling 'gross' or 'huge' instead of 'full' or 'satisfied'
- Wearing only loose-fitting clothes – due to negative body image, hiding weight loss, extreme discomfort due to feeling 'fat'
- Feeling guilty for eating, believing that one doesn't deserve to eat
- Ritualistic eating patterns

to get in touch with her body in a safe, non-judgmental way. It is common for those who suffer from eating disorders to be disembodied in the sense that they retreat into their minds to escape emotional pain and physiological discomfort. Many patients describe feeling 'safer' in their heads than in their bodies. Art therapy can also be an effective vehicle for exploring and healing body-image distortion/disparagement and self-esteem.

In many ways, experiential approaches enable the individual to express what is unspeakable because they can't find the language, the material is not conscious or the information is too terrifying to confront directly. What they can't say out loud, they may be able to draw, image, express in free-association writing or release in movement. These therapies offer creative ways to explore new possibilities for thinking and to access buried emotions. In addition, when tailored to the individual, they can capitalize on her creative talents and help to enhance self-esteem.

# Common psychological themes

While every patient brings a unique set of circumstances to individual psychotherapy, there are common psychological themes which emerge, including:

- low self-esteem and the need to acquire a positive sense of self
- an exploration of personal values including the meaning, advantages and disadvantages attached to eating-disorder symptoms
- depression and suicidality
- cognitive distortions and obsessional thinking
- interpersonal relationships
- the inability to recognize interoceptive cues such as hunger and satiety (fullness) and internal feeling states, especially anger, loneliness, anxiety, guilt and shame
- control issues, including the rigidity and overcontrol common in anorexia nervosa and the impulsivity and dyscontrol more frequently found in bulimia nervosa
- body-image distortion/disparagement: it is essential that specific body-image interventions be employed in treatment programs. Research has shown that risk for developing an eating disorder is best predicted by body-image disturbances and that relapse is often related to failure to address these issues in therapy (Rosen, 1996). While consciousness-raising through psychoeducational materials is a positive step, most patients need specific strategies to deal with negative body image. Interventions which combine guided imagery

with movement therapy (Hutchinson, 1994) or cognitive-behavioral techniques and guided imagery (Kearney-Cooke and Striegel-Moore, 1997)
have proven to be helpful
- food abuse and self-starvation as a reaction to traumatic stress. This includes
symptoms of emotional numbing, panic attacks, dissociation and self-
injury.

The success of any approach to individual psychotherapy depends on the
patient's acknowledgment of her eating disorder and her willingness to engage
in the therapeutic process. In order to enhance motivation for change, Vitousek
and Watson (1998) advocate the Socratic method which uses a series of hypo-
thetical, third-person questions designed to help patients explore information
and draw their own conclusions. Unlike highly interpretive approaches where
the therapist is the expert and tells the patient how it is, the Socratic method
encourages the patient to take the lead in making connection. This style is used
in the cognitive-behavioral approach. The emphasis is on collaboration, openness, patience, individual discovery and joint systematic inquiry. The authors
emphasize four themes deemed crucial in engaging reluctant individuals with
eating disorders. These include the provision of psychoeducational materials,
an examination of the advantages and disadvantages of symptoms, an exploration of personal values and the explicit use of experimental ('Let's try this out
and see what happens') strategies. These themes are also core features of a
patient-centered approach to individual treatment.

# Group psychotherapy

Research on group psychotherapy for eating disorders has focussed primarily on
bulimia nervosa since the early 1980s when this disorder was first classified as a
diagnostic entity separate from anorexia nervosa. As a result, most of the literature on group treatment is specific to bulimia nervosa and many authors actually
recommend excluding individuals suffering from anorexia nervosa from groups.
The reasons for this are discussed in terms of cautions and contraindications for
group therapy later in this section. Group formats are considered to be both cost-
and time-effective. They have become the major treatment components in many
day treatment and partial hospitalization programs where patients suffering
from both anorexia nervosa and bulimia nervosa are represented.

The variety of approaches to group treatment can be divided into two general
types; didactic approaches and interactional approaches. Didactic approaches
concentrate on imparting information and teaching specific skills such as assertion, normalization of eating patterns/nutrition counseling and stress management. These groups tend to be short-term and psychoeducational in nature and
may deal with several issues or target a single aspect of eating disorders such

as body image and self-esteem. Interactional approaches are insight-oriented, longer-term and tend to focus more on underlying psychological and inter-personal issues than on the management of eating, weight and physiological symptoms (Polivy and Federoff, 1997). Psychodynamic group therapy exempli-fies this approach.

Cognitive-behavioral approaches are semi-structured and directive in format. Techniques used are similar to those described in the section on individual psy-chotherapy. Frequently used techniques include self-monitoring (of food intake, binge/purge episodes, trigger emotions, etc.), psychoeducation, assertion train-ing, relaxation training and cognitive-restructuring.

Groups such as Overeaters Anonymous (OA) are based on the addiction model. An addictions orientation views eating disorders as variants of substance abuse disorders. The focus is on the 'addictive personality' and the individual's relationship with food is seen as an addiction. Like Alcoholics Anonymous (AA) where abstinence from alcohol is demanded, OA groups demand abstinence from binge eating, or in some cases, avoidance of trigger foods such as chocolate or refined sugar. According to Polivy and Federoff (1997), addiction models of treatment are not widely advocated by the therapeutic community. There are several reasons for this (Wilson, 1991). First, treatments for substance abuse are based on an abstinence model. For those who struggle with eating disorders, abstinence from certain foods promotes dieting, and dieting tends to intensify self-starvation and exacerbate binge eating in eating disorders. Second, the addictions model does not address several core clinical features of eating disor-ders including irrational ideas about food and weight, body-image disturbance and psychobiological connections between self-starvation and eating disorders. Third, the difficulties encountered by patients with eating disorders go beyond dieting and binge eating; the addictions model fails to address issues like perso-nal identity, excessive needs for control, emotional sensitivity, etc. Finally, the addictions model promotes a uniformity myth about anorexia nervosa, bulimia nervosa and binge-eating disorder and ignores differences among the various eating disorders (Polivy and Federoff, 1997).

In a recent review of the factors influencing the effectiveness of group psy-chotherapy for bulimia nervosa, McKisack and Waller (1997) concluded that there was no obvious advantage to any specific theoretical approach to group treatment. Better outcome was, however, associated with longer, more inten-sively scheduled groups and the addition of other treatment components; for example, individual work. Currently, a blend of cognitive–behavioral and inter-actional approaches is being advocated as the most efficacious because it addresses personal and interpersonal issues in combination with cognitive dis-tortions and normalization of eating patterns.

There are several potential advantages to group psychotherapy in the treat-ment of eating disorders. Groups offer a reduction in social isolation and aliena-tion. Hope is instilled when patients see other group members managing their distress and making progress toward recovery. In addition, individuals feel less alone as they hear others relate their personal histories and current struggles with their eating disorder. This plus the empathic responses of other group members can decrease feelings of shame and help release suppressed emotions. Finally, groups provide a context for learning and practising interpersonal skills and healing relational wounds. The views of patients themselves appear to support the efficacy of group treatment. In a study conducted by Rorty *et al.* (1993), contact with other sufferers was rated as one of the most helpful treatment-related experiences. In addition, 76% of the women who attended group therapy were satisfied with the treatment.

While research on practical guidelines for conducting group psychotherapy in the treatment of eating disorders is still in its infancy, some cautions and contraindications are emerging. Group treatment may be contraindicated for patients struggling with personality disorders, severe depression, high suicide risk, substance abuse, self-harm behaviors and extreme shyness (Kaplan and Olmsted, 1997; Polivy and Federoff, 1997). One important concern expressed by clinicians and attested to by patients is that group members may teach each other new weight-loss techniques and unhealthy thought patterns or foster a heightened competition with each other for being the thinnest. If such issues are not directly addressed in the group, an overidentification with the eating disorder as defining one's identity can develop. For these reasons, some group therapists advocate against group therapy for anorexia nervosa patients who evidence strong denial and resistance to change.

With these cautions in mind, group psychotherapy appears to be well-received by the patients themselves when the group is run by competent leaders experienced in the treatment of eating disorders. In their evaluations of a group which focussed on the development of coping strategies for recovery from bulimia nervosa, participants offered the following reactions:

> 'I'm so glad other group members talked about their anger. I always thought there was something wrong with me for feeling so angry. Now I know that it's just a normal emotion that everyone feels. I think I've been pushing it down with food. It's like now I have permission to really speak out about it.'
>
> 'I learned that I'm not alone. Not only did I learn things from other members of the group who are farther ahead than me, it also makes me feel good to know that I can help others and that they really value my personal opinions.'
>
> 'There were other members of the group I could identify with. That really helped me. I'm not sure what it was but I think that listening to them made me feel less strange about myself.'

Support groups are an important adjunct to professionally managed individual and group treatments. In general, there is little or no cost incurred and the group is held in a non-therapeutic setting. These groups may be run by a professional or non-professional and attendance is not usually mandatory. Depending on an individual's area of expertise, those run by a professional often include some skills teaching in the areas of enhancing self-esteem, becoming more assertive, managing stress or normalizing eating patterns. Educational videos, speakers and access to articles and books may be offered. The strength of support groups lies in the offering of contact, acceptance, encouragement and the provision of referral and informational resources. Family support groups can also be extremely helpful to parents and significant others who live with sufferers. The sharing of stories and coping strategies with other families is often comforting, helps to reduce stress and instills hope.

Hall and Cohn (1999) have provided a basic framework for forming a support group run by individuals struggling with bulimia nervosa. The guidelines provide suggestions on how to advertise the group, discussion topics, rotational assignments of facilitator, time-keeper and gripe-control monitor and how to begin and end meetings. Finally, several support groups are offered on the internet.

# Family therapy

*Dermot J Hurley*

As the emphasis of this book is primarily on the outpatient management of young persons with eating disorders, the following discussion deals with situations where a family presents for the first time with an eating disorder, or where the family is in outpatient treatment over a period of time, often with a number of relapses and readmissions to hospital. In the latter case it is likely that a number of key professionals are involved in the treatment process, which means that a significant level of co-ordination between professionals is necessary if iatrogenic effects are to be avoided. If the young person is hospitalized, then the focus of the treatment is invariably on her as an individual, and involves a combination of medical, nursing, psychiatric and psychosocial interventions aimed at refeeding and weight restoration. However, the support of the family in this phase of treatment is critical, and many problems can be avoided by involving the family in key decisions that impact on the treatment process. It is essential that the family clearly understands the process as well as the goals of treatment. Similarly, the treatment team needs to listen to the family and to understand the uniqueness of their experience of living with the disorder. Programs vary with respect to the degree of involvement of family members, with some advocating minimal involvement of the parents in the early stages of inpatient treatment of an adolescent with an eating disorder. Other programs are more inclusive and assign a family therapist to work with the family immediately on admission of the patient.

From the outset the clinician must be sensitive to the ongoing struggle in the family over the issue of food and attempt to divert the discussion away from emotionally charged areas early on in the interview. If the client has attained an inpatient status, much of the initial work of the family therapist is to link the family and the inpatient team in developing a working therapeutic alliance. Additionally, the family therapist must assess the contribution of the family to the development and maintenance of the disorder, and determine how best to engage the family in the treatment process. Families with eating disorders have two kinds of counseling needs. The first is family psychoeducation and the second is family therapy. A primary issue is to distinguish between the role of family psychoeducation and that of family therapy in resolving issues presented by families with eating disorders. Typically, family psychoeducation involves various professionals who offer perspectives on nutrition, health and eating disorders. A health practitioner and a nutritionist (either working separately or together) are key players in this discussion, and the family are made aware of the ramifications of aberrant nutrition and poor eating habits on the growth and development of the individual. Many related issues are discussed, including lifestyle, meal planning and preparation, physical and social activities, school, work etc., depending on the stage of development of the individual affected. Myths and distortions are openly discussed, and the goals of treatment are outlined with the family. It is an opportunity for the family to voice their concerns and for the team to get to know more about the family and its unique circumstances. If a target weight is set for the identified patient, and the 'contract' is relatively straightforward, the clinician can move ahead and discuss with the family whether other health professionals or resources should be involved.

The decision to involve a psychologist/psychotherapist and a family therapist should be mutual, ensuring that a sense of collaboration is fostered from the beginning. A feeling of empowerment is important for the family with an eating-disordered individual as it sets the stage for collaborative effort and family involvement in treatment. At the end of the first meeting an agreement can usually be reached and a copy of the treatment contract circulated to the family and to the professionals involved. Clearly, not all family members will agree to the treatment plan, and it is usual for the person with anorexia nervosa to disagree with the goal of weight gain. Reframing the issue as 'developing good eating habits' or 'maintaining a healthy lifestyle' can ameliorate to some extent the focus on negative aspects of the problem. Acknowledging the lone dissenting voice (usually the patient) and her feelings on the issue of treatment is a first step in developing some co-operation on treatment goals. Family collaboration is a key issue from the beginning of treatment, and every effort is made to avoid labeling the family as the problem or the person suffering from the illness.

# Issues in beginning family therapy

Typically, parents and siblings of a young person with an eating disorder are most anxious for guidance in how to deal with some of the problems inherent in living with a person with an eating disorder. If the young person is 19 or younger and living at home, a standard family treatment can be offered that is routinely used with this population (Dare *et al.*, 1990). The Maudsley group in London, UK, combines two family therapy approaches in dealing with eating disorders (Dare and Eisler, 1997). The first is a problem-solving approach directed specifically at the symptoms. The second is a systems approach which invites family members to consider the interconnectedness of their behavior and feelings as they relate to the eating disorder. The problem-solving approach focuses on the immediate issues at hand and the intervention is aimed at the parents' taking charge of their child's eating behavior. This aspect of treatment has much in common with Minuchin *et al.*'s (1978) structural family therapy approach. The process works in three distinct phases. The first involves refeeding the client, the second focuses on the renegotiation of new family patterns and the third is a termination phase when healthy weight has been resumed. This approach has been shown to be affective with adolescent eating-disordered clients and good results are maintained at the five-year follow-up mark (Eisler *et al.*, 1997). For adults with severe anorexia nervosa, inpatient staff usually take the parental role in the refeeding process.

If the person is over 19 and living away from home, a different type of family treatment can be offered as an adjunct to individual therapy, which is usually the treatment of choice. Family therapy with this older population has generally not received the same kind of research efficacy that is noted for the younger population, though clinically, family-therapy interventions have had quite positive outcomes in selected cases of young adults and their families. Generally, it is the rule that when a young person is residing at home, or where the affected individual is a spouse, other family members are invited to attend family sessions on a routine basis.

From the onset, the clinician must be sensitive to the ongoing struggle in the family over the issue of food and attempt to divert the discussion away from emotionally charged areas early on in the interview. If the patient has attained an inpatient status, much of the initial work of the family therapist is aimed at connecting the family and the inpatient team in developing a working therapeutic alliance. Additionally, the family therapist must assess the contribution of the family to the development and maintenance of the disorder, and determine how best to engage the family in the treatment process.

Initially, a family needs to vent their feelings and talk about their fears for the safety of the person living with an eating disorder. It is important for them to know that the treatment team understands the often bizarre situation that they're living in. It is often a relief to hear that there are many other families in the same predicament and to hear anecdotes of how other families have dealt with similar problems. The family may describe themselves as prisoners in their own home, or as 'living with a food tyrant', who controls most of what happens in the home. The family therapist must be sensitive to descriptions of the patient that further diminish their personhood, and must balance his or her inquiry with questions pertaining to areas of competence and resilience in the individual.

Narrative therapy encourages the separation of the person from the problem, by labeling the eating disorder, not the person, as 'the problem' (White and Epston, 1990). The narrative approach allows for new ideas and possibilities to emerge, and invites a reauthoring of the individual's life and relationships. In externalizing the disorder in this way, the affected individual comes to see herself as a person struggling to overcome the oppression of anorexia nervosa or bulimia nervosa, rather than the one who is to blame for the disorder.

The task of the family therapist is to access important information without scapegoating the eating-disordered individual, or allowing the affect in the session to get out of control. The experience of the person suffering with an eating disorder is critical information, and allows for some balance to be achieved in the session between the family's concerns and the emotional conflicts of the identified client. Care should also be taken to inquire about other areas of family functioning, particularly areas of strength and competence which are often overshadowed by the disorder.

It is particularly important for the family to understand the effects of severe malnutrition and to distinguish the starvation effects of the disorder from the personality characteristics of the individual. The family needs to appreciate that the young person may be clinically depressed or suffering from an obsessive–compulsive disorder (OCD) as a consequence of or co-morbid with the eating disorder. Often the affected person is extremely socially isolated from their peer group, and can become even more emotionally isolated in the family as a consequence of the disorder. It is extremely distressing for the family not to know how to help during a full-blown anorectic or bulimic episode, and they often report feeling completely helpless at these times.

There are other practical impacts that families have to deal with, such as heat regulation in the home as a consequence of hypothermia experienced by the person with anorexia nervosa. Trivial as it may seem, other family members may overheat as a result of the furnace thermostat being kept on high, which ironically comes to mirror the emotional climate in the family. Space utilization is also a key issue as the anorectic or bulimic person suffering from a food phobia/addiction may come to view the kitchen as their own private property. Meal times are typically a problem for the family, while the kitchen area, and the refrigerator in particular, are described as a 'disaster zone' or 'nightmare'. Issues related to cleanliness, hygiene and storage of food are frequently on the agenda for family therapy sessions. Bathroom use is also an area of conflict as the person with an eating disorder may spend a disproportionate amount of time in the bathroom. Often, a person suffering with anorexia nervosa is affected by noise, at times even the sound of a human voice, which has an impact on other family members who may not appreciate this acoustic sensitivity. They may misinterpret this sensitivity as one more area of family living which is being controlled by anorexia nervosa or bulimia nervosa.

Lastly, there are additional financial costs to living with an eating disorder, not just in terms of the cost of food which can be considerable (it is frequently wasted in the case of anorexia nervosa and consumed in large quantities in the case of bulimia nervosa), but in terms of additional professional services which may not be covered by regular medical insurance.

# Family assessment

The main issue in a family assessment is to get information from the family about how they are currently functioning, how they are affected by the disorder and how they contribute to the maintenance of the problem, if indeed they do.

At the same time, the family therapist is looking for opportunities to be helpful, and may suggest areas for intervention immediately following the first meeting. As in any family assessment, a balance is maintained between past and present. However, in families with an eating disorder it is critical to intervene early in family communications that trigger conflict (Le Grange 1999), and to identify 'problem-maintaining patterns' in which symptoms are embedded.

There are a number of family assessment protocols that can be utilized with families, and a model of a family assessment has been described by Shekter-Wolfson and Woodside (1990) specifically for families with eating-disordered adolescents. They follow the American Psychiatric Association treatment guidelines for eating disorders which strongly recommend a family assessment for clients who are living at home with their parents. Such an assessment should have the following components:

- identifying data
- current family situation
- family's knowledge about the eating disorder
- family's theory about the origin of the eating disorder
- family's efforts to help the identified client
- family's eating habits
- family's attitude to weight and shape.

(Shekter-Wolfson and Woodside, 1990)

In assessing families with eating disorders, other areas of equal importance would include:

- organizing impact of the symptoms on the family
- areas of family life not affected by the disorder
- family strengths and competencies
- identified patients perceptions of family influences
- family-therapeutic system linkages

The family therapist's assumptions about eating disorders are an important aspect of treating eating-disordered families. Assumptions about client problems orient the therapist toward a particular therapeutic posture which can limit or enhance the therapeutic process (Tomm, 1987). Eating disorders often invite reductionistic thinking and linear assumptions. Because these disorders are difficult to treat and frustrating for therapist and client, there is a tendency to pathologize and blame the client or family for the problem. Since these emotional attitudes are couched in clinical language they have a ring of authenticity when spoken. If the assumptions that underlie the emotional attitudes remain unexamined they will affect the course and outcome of therapy. How a family therapist thinks and acts are important determinants of successful therapy.

The following therapeutic orientation to families with eating disorders has been found to be helpful in working with adolescent clients and their families:

- respect for family members and their perception of events
- acceptance without blame of the family's predicament
- future rather than past orientation
- openness to the unique experience of the family and their circumstances
- non-assumptive stance about past treatment failures.

# Engaging the family in the therapeutic process

Engaging the whole family in the treatment process is a critical first step in working with eating-disordered families. That is not to suggest that all family members must attend all sessions or that the therapist cannot meet individually with various family members. The main point is that the therapist maintains a family focus and invites members to attend sessions without coercion. With younger eating-disordered clients it is crucial to involve both parents and to develop a working alliance with them, whether they are living together or apart.

The scope of the book does not allow for an in-depth discussion of family therapy with the divorced members. However, it is important to remember that there are important similarities and differences related to eating patterns in each home. Frequently, the family therapist is polarized from the beginning by parents who are in conflict, and every attempt is made to not be drawn in on one side or the other. This will be the first issue for the family therapist to deal with prior to establishing a workable treatment contract.

It is important to explain how family therapy works, and for the therapist to develop a clear understanding with the family about how sessions will proceed. Initially, the young person may not wish to be part of treatment and may challenge the whole idea of a family focus. The issue here is not to engage in a power struggle but to proceed with family therapy with those members most willing to come.

The initial session is an opportunity to correct misperceptions, clarify misunderstandings and hear the frustration and concern of the family. A subsequent goal is to assess the impact of the disorder on the family, as well as the impact of the family on the disorder. The therapist's job is to try and get the family to be more solution-focused and engaged in the process of therapy (de Shazer, 1982). A good deal of conflict may be generated in these sessions and the family therapist must be able to sort out what is particularly relevant to the problems presented by the family.

The session goes beyond simple information sharing, and invites the family to discuss issues that arise with the treatment team's management of the individual patient. Frequently, the family is confused about aspects of the treatment strategy, and their misunderstanding may reveal a lack of integration and co-ordination between various treatment providers in the treatment system. For instance, a family may be very concerned about their daughter's restrictive eating and excessive exercise which is keeping her weight at a critical level. The psychotherapist on the other hand may be less concerned about her eating behavior, but more interested in evidence of her growing autonomy. While supporting the young person in taking responsibility for her own nutrition, they may not consider the disruptive impact her current eating pattern is having on the family.

In working with eating-disordered families, it is not unusual to find that information is distorted or incomplete. Anorexia nervosa and bulimia nervosa can affect the cognitive process of all family members and there is a high level of emotional arousal and contagion in the family. The family may appear to have lost a sense of direction and purpose. To the professional, it may seem as if no one is 'in charge' of the family, and that the anorexia nervosa or bulimia nervosa is 'driving the system' and creating its own unique impact on the individuals concerned. The problem is said at this stage to be organizing the system.

'Problem organizing systems' have been described elsewhere, and are not unique to anorexia nervosa or bulimia nervosa (Anderson and Goolishan, 1988). However, eating disorders have a particular type of organizing impact that limit and constrain options when attempts are made to change the system.

Eating disorders are resistant to change and appear to take on a 'life of their own' in families where the primary focus over many years is the eating problem. A family may have become acclimatized to such an extent that they no longer have a picture of what normal family life is or should be. They have forgotten how they were prior to the disorder, and have adapted and accommodated to the demands of the eating disorder, to such an extent that the presenting situation vis à vis food can be truly bizarre. One family presented their anorectic daughter with three different choices for dinner each evening, and additionally would rush out and purchase fast food on a whim if she was not satisfied with the food that they had prepared for her.

There are a number of key roles that a family therapist plays in working with families with an eating disorder. These are as follows:

- lowering the overall level of conflict and anxiety in the family
- interrupting circular processes in which the symptom is embedded, and working with family members to disengage from the problem
- clarifying individual perceptions, thoughts, feelings and actions
- inviting alternative constructions of the problem and alternative views of the person
- acting as a catalyst for the pooling of knowledge, skills and resources at the individual, family, team and community levels.

Ownership of the problem by the identified client is a key issue in treating families with eating disorders, as the family may invest more time and energy in finding a solution than the person themselves. The young person must reclaim their own body and develop a sense of mastery in interpersonal relationships. In time, the intense relationship with the body will hopefully be given up for true assertion and independence. The family therapist must remain focused on the strengths of the family and desired outcomes. The goal is to engage the family in change strategies without further scapegoating the individual client. The family therapist maintains a systemic orientation and utilizes the input of all family members. Siblings are often angry and resentful about the amount of attention the affected individual is receiving from the parents. They may also feel that the parents are ineffective and indulging the young person and their problem. Many of these feelings need to be acknowledged in family sessions and resolved if possible. The inclusion of siblings can be extremely productive in family therapy sessions. One nine-year-old sister of a 13-year-old girl with anorexia nervosa offered the following advice in a family therapy session:

- eat well (not low-fat)
- focus on good things, not bad
- don't count calories in food
- don't keep on weighing yourself.

In essence, this nine-year-old summarized the main treatment issues for her sister, i.e. the importance of normal eating, negative cognitions and obsessive–compulsive patterns of behavior. Such contributions from family members may have a profound impact on the affected individual.

The family therapist helps create a climate of encouragement and realistic hope, while at the same time attending to ongoing conflict in the family. Helping the family to change dysfunctional patterns of interaction that maintain the symptoms is the number one priority. The family therapist may be aware of the possibility of deeper underlying issues that he or she may or may not be addressing in a particular session. The focus on more dynamic family issues may not be possible or advisable until a pattern of normal eating has resumed (Shekter-Wolfson *et al.*, 1997) The family needs time to develop trust in the therapist in order to make the changes necessary to sustain their recovery and avoid relapse. Finally, working through the inevitable losses brought about by these disorders and helping the family come to terms with the changes that have taken place in their life should occur prior to termination.

# Nutritional management through recovery

*Nancy E Strange*

Improvement of nutritional status is of the utmost importance in order for persons suffering from eating disorders to be able to benefit from therapy. In cases where physical health has been extremely compromised, hospitalization will be necessary, and in some cases more extreme measures of refeeding, such as elemental (tube) or total parenteral nutrition (TPN) may be required. As our focus is ambulatory care of individuals suffering from eating disorders, these two methods of restoring nutritional status will not be discussed.

Once the nutritional assessment is complete and nutritional intervention is about to begin, the patient and the dietitian will need to discuss the readiness of the patient to make changes in her eating behaviors. It is important to realize that change in eating patterns and consequent improvement of nutritional status will only occur when the individual is ready. Any changes that take place as a result of threats or other methods of coercion will be short-lived.

In some cases, many discussions will need to take place before the person suffering from an eating disorder will make the decision to commit to improving her eating habits. It is incredibly important for the dietitian to realize that this person will be giving up behaviors that have been her coping methods for quite some time and she may feel very insecure about doing this.

# Goal setting

Once the decision has been made, goal setting may begin. Again, it is important to emphasize that the goals must be those of the person suffering from the eating disorder in order for there to be incentive to work toward those goals.

Three main goals that are most common will be discussed here. They are:

- normalization of eating habits
- meeting nutritional needs
- specific weight goals.

Normalization of eating habits will have different meanings for different people. Looking at the patient's premorbid eating patterns is a good place to start. Often, persons suffering from eating disorders will say that they have forgotten what normal eating is. Normal eating habits are not necessarily three balanced meals daily at approximately the same times each day. Most people with normal eating habits do not fit this pattern. However, most people with normal eating habits do eat anywhere from three to five times during waking hours. Normal eating habits are flexible. They allow you to consume enough of each type of food daily to meet your nutritional needs. Normal eating habits do not call attention to yourself. Normal eating habits allow you to maintain a healthy weight without feeling constantly hungry. Normal eating habits permit you to eat all foods, so that obsessions about foods and binge eating do not occur. Eating normally means eating in response to hunger. Being able to eat normally is essential in order for recovery to occur.

Meeting nutritional needs implies that the person will be able in a typical day to consume enough different types of foods (solids and liquids), in sufficient quantities to meet all macro (protein, fat, carbohydrate and energy) and micro (vitamins, minerals, fluid and fibre) nutrient requirements as established by the American Recommended Daily Allowance (RDA) or the Canadian Recommended Nutrient Intake (RNI). These are the quantities of nutrients deemed to be necessary to promote good health and permit normal healthy functioning of the body.

Weight goals indicate a necessity to eventually achieve and maintain a healthy weight that will allow the body to function normally. For an adolescent who has still not finished her linear growth, this means a weight where linear growth will recommence. An adult who is finished growing will be able to mark this weight as one where her normal menstrual cycle resumes. It is important to note that sometimes normal menstrual cycles do not return until the individual has been at a healthy weight for about six months. A healthy weight for an individual is typically that which is calculated as her ideal weight. However, it must be kept in mind that a healthy weight at which a person may eat normally, meet her nutritional needs and resume normal menstrual function could be anywhere between 90% and 120% of that which has been designated as ideal for her.

# Steps in nutritional counseling

Nutrition counseling for a person suffering from an eating disorder is multi-faceted. It involves all the many aspects of behavior change around eating.

# Discussion of macro and micro nutrients

It is usually effective to start off with several sessions of nutrition education, as these are non-threatening to the person with the eating disorder. They are simply information-giving discussions regarding the nutritional values of foods and the nutritional needs of people at particular stages of life. Typically, persons suffering from eating disorders are very interested in this information, so these sessions are helpful in creating a comfortable and non-threatening relationship with the dietitian. The topics that should be covered in these meetings include discussions of all nutrient groups, i.e. proteins, fats, carbohydrates, water, the most significant vitamins and minerals and fibre (Hsu *et al.*, 1992). These discussions should include functions, sources and specific requirements of these various nutrients. It is most effective if the focus is on nutrition to promote good health and enjoyment of good food. It is important to note that although this part of the nutrition counseling which is specifically the nutrition education is very important and essential, it is probably the smallest component and will take the least time.

# Dealing with cognitive disorders

The time-consuming portions of the nutrition counseling involve facing and working on gradually changing the harmful eating patterns that have become established during the eating disorder. The dietitian has a responsibility to help the person to challenge and eventually change her cognitive distortions regarding food, weight and body image.

The dietitian must be aware that a behavior change is a process and not an event. It will take a long time and involve many small steps to go from disordered eating to normal eating. Challenging distorted beliefs begins early in the nutritional management process and continues throughout the entire recovery period. It is helpful for the dietitian and all therapists working with the individual suffering from an eating disorder to have a good comprehension of the functions of these cognitive distortions for the individual. Reiff and Lampson Reiff (1992) in their book *Eating Disorders: nutrition therapy in the recovery process*, describe the functions of cognitive disorders in the following manner. Firstly, they give the person a sense of control. If, for example, she believes that dairy products are fattening and she does not consume dairy products, she feels strong and in control. Secondly, they give her a sense of identity. To some persons suffering from eating disorders, especially those with anorexia nervosa, the way they eat becomes equated with who they are. It is what makes them special. 'Everyone knows I don't use dairy products'. Thirdly, they are necessary for her to perpetuate her behavior. They have become a coping mechanism for dealing with her feelings and fears about life. If she changes her beliefs so that they are more healthy, she will no longer be able to rationalize her behavior. Lastly, they become a way to justify her behavior to other people. 'If I eat dairy products I feel sick' or 'I can't eat foods that have fat in them because they disagree with me'.

Reiff and Lampson Reiff (1992) recommend specific steps to address distorted beliefs, which include:

- acknowledging that the person with the eating disorder makes the rules regarding her behaviors, and explaining that you believe she taught herself to think in certain ways as she developed the eating disorder
- presenting the truth as a statement of fact, and clarifying the consequences of acting upon her beliefs vs acting upon what is true
- describing how you would feel if she were to change her beliefs, and assuring her that you would not see that as failure on her part or winning on your part, but rather as a sign of growth and change that will help her get well.

The following case study illustrates how the above recommendations can work.

### Case study
Sheila was a 13-year-old who had the distorted belief that to consume any fat was bad and would lead to rapid weight gain. She had seen many advertisements on TV, denigrating fat while promoting fat-free products, during the early stages of her eating disorder. Thus, she had taken this to the extreme and done her best to eliminate all fat from her diet. When beginning nutrition intervention, this young lady was quite emaciated and had very dry, scaly skin. She was assured that she was the one in control of deciding her food intake, but it was pointed out to her that she had taught herself to think that all fat was bad, because of her strong desire to lose weight. The 'truth' was presented to her that fat is an essential nutrient for many body processes. The role of essential fatty acids in promoting healthy

skin was discussed. Another 'truth' presented was that a reasonable amount of fat in the diet would not promote excessive weight gain. It was pointed out that the media promotion of a lower-fat diet is aimed at people who have a tendency to consume an unbalanced diet with too large a proportion of the energy coming from one nutrient. It was also explained that the decision to include some fat would be hers and that it would not represent her giving up control, but rather making a positive step towards restoring her health and smooth, healthy skin. Sheila decided to allow herself a small amount of fat, mostly because she was very distressed about the appearance of her skin. Within three weeks she could see an improvement in her skin, even though the weight gain in that time period was quite small. She was pleased, and had made a positive step towards eliminating one cognitive distortion. Each time a distorted belief is challenged and a change in behavior takes place, even if it is a small change, it represents a step along the road to recovery.

# Recommended energy intake

An important issue in the refeeding process is the recommended energy (calorie) intake. The recommended energy intake will vary throughout the recovery process. This is because of the effects of starvation and refeeding on metabolic rate. When an individual dramatically reduces her caloric intake to lose weight, the metabolic rate begins to slow and hits bottom in 3–7 weeks (Kahm, 1994). Therefore, initial energy recommendations will be lower, i.e. 1200 calories will likely promote weight gain in the early stages when metabolic rate is low. However, after a small weight gain of two to three kgs, this energy intake will only maintain weight. Eventually, weight will again be lost at this calorie level because the metabolic rate will start to increase. Energy needs will continue to increase as weight is gained and normal metabolic rate is restored. The slowing of the metabolic rate is a great source of anxiety for individuals with anorexia nervosa. They tend to feel caught between a rock and a hard place. If they increase their food intake they will gain weight, even if they are still eating less than 'normal', because of their lower metabolic rate; however, increasing their intake is the only way to get their metabolic rate back to normal.

Total energy needs are quite variable within the population. We have specific guidelines for recommended energy intakes at different ages and stages of life. However, there is still great variability. A reasonably accurate assessment of the individual's caloric intake prior to the eating disorder is helpful when doing an initial assessment of energy needs. As refeeding takes place and weight is gained, caloric needs will continue to increase, and may go as high as 3500 calories a day to promote weight gain. However, once healthy weight is restored, the person who required 3500 calories to achieve that weight may be able to maintain it on approximately 2200–2400 calories a day. During the refeeding process, when the individual is slowly gaining weight and her metabolic rate is slowly returning to normal, there will be setbacks where the person has made a good effort to eat but weight is actually lost. It is very helpful at this time to point out to the individual that there is a bright side to this 'setback' (Beaumont *et al.*, 1997). It proves that her metabolic rate is improving and that really is a very good sign, because it will eventually allow her to eat normally and enjoy food with much less fear of weight gain.

# Eating in response to hunger

Eating in response to hunger is a process that must be relearned. It is not that persons suffering from eating disorders do not experience hunger. As mentioned in Chapter 1, the term anorexia nervosa is a misnomer. One young lady told the writer that she was constantly hungry, and that she had to fight that hunger with all her strength in order not to give in to it. Coffee, cigarettes, diet pop and other very low-calorie items are used to dull the hunger pangs. Most people with anorexia nervosa are aware of their hunger but choose to disregard it whenever possible. Some individuals with eating disorders actually take pleasure in the hunger sensations, especially in the early stages of their eating disorders, because these feelings signal to them they are losing weight and they are 'in control'.

Hunger involves a rather complex interplay amongst several factors; blood levels of glucagon in collaboration with insulin, stomach contents, the individual's current weight in relationship with ideal weight or usual weight and the body's need for energy-containing foods and specific essential nutrients. Hunger may include thirst, a craving for carbohydrates, a craving for protein, a craving for fats and a desire for an adequate total number of calories to satisfy the needs of the body. When a person eats in a consistent manner, her body will develop a hunger pattern such that she will experience hunger at fairly predictable times during the day. A person who has developed an eating disorder will eat only when she tells herself it is permissible, and only those foods and amounts of foods that she classifies as acceptable. The body responds by intensifying the degree of hunger, thereby increasing obsessional thinking about food. The individual with an eating disorder then begins to distrust the hunger signals she is getting because her sense is that she is always hungry and if she gives in to these feelings she will totally lose control and not be able to stop eating. Often, it becomes necessary for the person suffering from an eating disorder to eat almost 'mechanically' at specified meal and snack times in order to create a hunger pattern that she will eventually be able to trust (Howard and Krug Porzelius, 1999).

There is a fairly wide variation in normal hunger patterns. Some of the factors that are responsible for specific hunger patterns include school schedule, work schedule, sleep patterns, regularity of food-intake patterns, biological parameters, i.e. blood sugar level, and cultural expectations. Part of the nutrition management must be helping the individual with an eating disorder to re-establish her hunger patterns based on her own schedule. This involves discussing with the individual exactly what her usual daily routine consists of, and giving her guidelines to follow as to when her meals and snacks should be, in addition to quantities and types of foods to include. It may take several weeks or even months before the individual will begin to respond to her new hunger patterns.

# Barriers to normal eating

In addition to the already mentioned issues such as cognitive distortions regarding food and eating, and fear of losing control, there are also some physiological 'barriers' to normal eating that must be addressed. These include early satiety and weight fluctuations, particularly in response to fluid or hydration shifts.

After a lengthy period of very low volume of food intake, it is not unusual for a person to experience some gastrointestinal abnormalities, such as delayed gastric emptying and decreased intestinal motility. These may produce a strong sense of stomach fullness, even abdominal discomfort and constipation. These gastrointestinal symptoms often interfere with the process of normalization of eating habits. The individual may feel that she cannot increase her intake of food at meals because she feels full so quickly. The poor bowel motility may be so concerning to her that she self-medicates with laxatives in order to experience relief. The result of this of course is often diarrhea which may lead to dehydration and electrolyte (particularly potassium) depletion. It is very important for the dietitian to acknowledge these problems and assist the person suffering from the eating disorder to understand why these symptoms are occurring and that they can gradually resolve through the process of improving her eating habits.

Early satiety necessitates six small meals daily, rather than three regular meals and three snacks for some individuals. Once they are tolerating the six small meals, they should be encouraged to gradually work at making three of the meals larger until they are close to normal size. It is usually helpful to make up a meal plan that specifies food groups and appropriate portion sizes. In the author's experience, the meal plan will be much more effectively used if the person with the eating disorder is actively involved in setting it up. There are some individuals who appear to prefer to have the meal plan made up for them by the dietitian. However, most do better if they have some ownership of the plan. After the standard meal plan is established, and the individual is following it with a reasonable degree of success, then a graduated program of increasing number or size of portions may be set up. It must be remembered that it may take weeks or even months for a motivated individual to achieve a degree of comfort with normal portion sizes.

Hydration shifts are responsible for some intense emotional responses in some persons suffering from eating disorders. The person will usually feel that she is getting fat because refeeding causes her to gain water weight. She may feel bloated and swollen. The individual with the eating disorder is typically dehydrated at the initiation of refeeding. A weight gain of one to three kgs over a few days is not uncommon as the body rehydrates. This may intensify the patient's distrust of food and also may spark some distrust of the dietitian. The dietitian can help at this point by explaining the hydration shifts in simple terms. Each human body has its own specific fluid volume, which it defends. An individual with anorexia nervosa becomes dehydrated due to restricted intake of both fluids and solids. The body stores carbohydrates with water; consequently, when carbohydrate intake is severely cut back the body will have less fluid on board, which is reflected by a lower weight on the scale. An individual with bulimia nervosa, who has been vomiting regularly will lose body fluid and electrolytes in the process. When these situations occur, the body will do whatever it needs to do to rectify the situation. When subjected to periods of fluid deprivation, the body's response is to retain more fluid than normal, almost as if it were 'preparing for a drought or famine'. For example, when a person suffering with anorexia nervosa begins to eat more normally (i.e. include more carbohydrates in her meals, and drink more liquids) her body will retain more water than usual until it is 'convinced' that fluids will be available on a regular basis again. At that point the extra fluid will be lost through urination. The individual with bulimia nervosa will notice a similar 'shift' and hold extra fluid for a few days until electrolyte levels are normal.

If the person with the eating disorder is reassured that the weight change is indeed water and not fat, and that this fluid retention is temporary, it may help her to continue with her recovery process rather than to sabotage her efforts in frustration. The individual suffering with an eating disorder tends to be very focused on the number on the scale, so this will be a very difficult and emotional issue and it will likely need to be explained more than once.

# Preoccupation with thoughts of food as a result of starvation

It is not uncommon for an individual suffering from an eating disorder to spend 80% or even more of her waking hours thinking about food and eating. In fact, many patients have described dreams in which they were eating 'forbidden foods', most commonly ice cream. It is not at all surprising that a person who is always hungry becomes preoccupied with thoughts of food. This is part of the body's normal survival mechanism. A case example is as follows.

**Case study**
Maureen was 15 years old when she began nutrition counseling for her eating disorder. She was 5′3″ tall and weighed 94 lbs. She had lost 23 lbs over a three-month period. She shared with the dietitian that she did feel a certain satisfaction with her weight, in that her initial goal had been 99 lbs. She said she wanted to improve her health and nutrition but not gain any weight. When asked if there were any issues related to her weight loss that were concerning to her, she cited two. As it turned out, the two were closely related. One concern was that her marks in school were dropping; marks that had previously been in the high 80s were now in the low 70s. The other was her decreasing ability to concentrate in school or when doing her homework, due to almost constant thoughts about food and eating. She indicated that she felt she had no control over this, and the harder she tried to concentrate, the more the thoughts of food intruded. It was explained to her that this was a totally natural process and it was her body's way of trying to give her the message that she needed to eat. She was also told that if she gradually improved her state of nutrition by eating in a non-restrictive way, these thoughts would gradually disappear. It was also explained to her that if she persisted with her current restrictive eating patterns, she was at a greater-than-normal risk of developing a problem with binge eating. Maureen wanted to be rid of these intrusive thoughts but the fear of increasing her body weight was overwhelming. As her level of self-esteem improved, and some personal issues were resolved, she allowed herself to increase her food intake. She now eats almost normally and her weight is 105 lbs. She is happy to report that although she thinks that thoughts about food still play a larger-than-normal role in her life, she is able to concentrate on her studies again and her grades are improving.

Once the body is completely renourished and weight is normal, preoccupation with thoughts of food usually subsides. However, it is important to remember that a person who has recovered from an eating disorder is still at greater risk from preoccupation with thoughts of food than a person who has never had an eating disorder.

# Social aspects of eating

Food and eating tend to be integral parts in many aspects of life. By no means can one think of food solely as a means of nourishing the body. Once the individual suffering from an eating disorder has made reasonable improvement in her nutritional status and is eating appropriate meals with a level of comfort, it is time to start working on dealing with the social aspects of eating. Despite achieving a healthy weight and meeting nutritional needs on a regular basis, an individual cannot be considered as 'recovered' if she continues to avoid social situations that revolve around food, or if she feels a need to 'control' such situations in order to take part.

In dealing with this aspect of the recovery process, it is helpful to initially engage the person recovering from an eating disorder in discussions regarding the social meanings of food in her particular family and situation. Starting back in infancy, where being fed when hungry provides the baby with a sense of physical comfort and safety, the relationship between food and emotions begins. Often, parents give their children 'treats' for 'being good' or bringing home a good report card. This tends to cause people to form an emotional response to food. Food is frequently used to express love. It is useful to list with the individual all the situations she can think of where food plays a role other than just that of nourishing the physical body. The list will likely include such occasions as birthdays, religious holidays, eating out, going to someone's home for dinner, dating and others. Many families have particular rituals that all members enjoy, such as routinely having pizza on Friday night as a treat. Once the list is complete, the process of sorting out the issues related to each situation can begin. The issues will be slightly different for those recovering from bulimia nervosa than for those dealing with the complications of anorexia nervosa. The concerns that tend to be cited by individuals with anorexia nervosa include: fear of unknown content of combination dishes, unknown caloric content of foods served, lack of control over meal timing, a sense of needing to starve all day in order to "save calories' for the special meal, and possible comments regarding her food intake by friends or family members. In addition to these concerns, the person recovering from bulimia fears that she may lose control and binge when confronted with appealing foods in a social situation.

Resuming normal eating in social situations will be one of the last stages of the recovering process and will likely take place very slowly, as the individual's level of confidence in her ability to succeed gradually improves. Several strategies for helping her to make the transition back to normal 'social' eating are discussed here.

If unknown caloric density of foods is a concern, the dietitian can help the individual learn to estimate the approximate caloric content of a variety of dishes. Although by this point in the recovery process it is preferable for the individual to be past the point of counting calories, stressful situations such as eating in a social context tend to cause reliance on some old habits such as calorie counting as a safety net. This is quite acceptable in the early stages, as it allows the individual a feeling of security.

As far as concern about the exact content of particular foods being served goes, the dietitian can again assist the individual to assume 'possible contents' of dishes. Preparation and discussion of a list of foods that evoke apprehension may be helpful. A discussion of her feelings about the taste and the level of enjoyment the food might provide should take place along with the discussion of possible ingredients, and the fears that these ingredients might evoke in the individual.

Fears of lack of control over meal timing are very much related to the rigidity that often comes along with eating disorders. Sometimes the fear is that they will become too hungry if they are forced to eat later than usual. For an individual recovering from anorexia nervosa this becomes physically very uncomfortable if she is not yet consistently consuming normal portions of food. She will have difficulty concentrating on the conversation because of her preoccupation with her sense of hunger. She is also worried that she may eat too much if she gets too hungry. For the person recovering from bulimia nervosa, the concern is that if the meal is later than usual she may lose control and binge. For both types of eating disorders the solution is the same. It is important for the individual to have a small snack such as a piece of fruit or a few crackers if the meal is going to be later than she is accustomed to. She will then be physically comfortable and able to participate in the conversation. Also, she will have a better control of her intake by not letting herself get overly hungry.

The sense of needing to starve all day in order to go out for dinner in the evening is a strong one and difficult to break. It is important for the dietitian to point out the risks inherent in this behavior. This type of behavior sets the person recovering from an eating disorder up to feel uncomfortable all day. It also will very likely lead to overeating when out, and possibly even binge eating. The importance of eating regularly throughout the day in order to maintain a sense of physical comfort and normal blood sugar levels should be explained. The individual then embarks on the evening out feeling in control, and knowing she will be able to eat appropriate quantities, and be less at risk of overeating.

Often persons who have suffered for a long period of time from an eating disorder, are uncomfortable with comments from well-meaning friends and relatives, when they see her eating normally again. Dealing with this issue can be tricky; however, in most cases it works best to confront it head on. The dietitian may encourage the patient to respond to family members or friends who comment on her eating, by telling them that although she knows they mean well, it is uncomfortable for her to have her eating habits commented on and she would prefer that they not do it.

Dealing with the social aspects of eating is extremely important in the overall recovery in order to prevent or correct the social isolation that can be very painful.

# Promotion of normal attitudes toward food

Normal attitudes toward food imply allowing oneself to enjoy food without thinking in terms of 'What will this do to my weight?'. It implies being able to eat when hungry, stop when satisfied, and to 'trust' food. In order for a person recovering from an eating disorder to truly achieve a normal attitude toward food, she must accept herself at a normal weight (Berg, 1996). She can never really be at peace with food if she continues to attempt to keep her body weight at an abnormally low level. It is, therefore, of the utmost importance that the nutritional counseling emphasizes good nutrition to promote good health and positive body image right from the start. This is very different from the distorted 'good nutrition to promote weight loss' emphasis that many persons suffering from eating disorders adopt. In order to 'pull together' all aspects of nutritional counseling, i.e. meeting nutritional needs, eating in response to hunger, dealing with cognitive distortions etc., it is extremely important to integrate work on positive body image and self-esteem. This is an area where the therapist and dietitian should collaborate in order to best serve the needs of the patient. It will be impossible for the individual recovering from an eating disorder to truly normalize her attitude toward eating until she is comfortable in her own body and accepts herself for who she is instead of always trying to improve herself.

Some of the ways in which the dietitian may help the individual along the path toward a normal attitude toward food, include making the following recommendations:

- physically relax your body just prior to eating a meal or snack
- practice thinking positive thoughts about the food being consumed, i.e. 'This really tastes good' or 'This will give me energy to get through the afternoon'
- allow yourself to really savor the flavors and textures of favorite foods
- when the meal or snack is completed, occupy your thoughts elsewhere, and move on with your day; do not continue to think about and analyse what you have eaten.

Typically, a person recovering from an eating disorder will feel a great sense of relief once she has truly normalized her attitude towards food.

# Specific guidelines for overcoming bulimic behavior or purging

Often a person suffering from bulimia nervosa is at or above her ideal weight. Despite this fact, it is important to keep in mind that she may very likely be malnourished depending on her specific food choices and the foods, both solids and liquids, that she actually retains. Therefore, it is essential to focus on meeting nutritional needs simultaneously with breaking the binge–purge cycle. It is quite common for an individual suffering from bulimia nervosa to alternate between periods of restricting and periods of bingeing and purging. It is important for the dietitian to help her to see the relationship between the restrictive eating and the bingeing and to explain how the restricting can actually 'trigger' the bingeing. Once again we find ourselves back to the theme of 'normalization' of eating habits, in order to cue the body that it is well cared-for and well-nourished. There are several steps that may be helpful for the recovery from bulimia nervosa that will be outlined here.

In the initial stages, it may be helpful for the person recovering from bulimia nervosa to follow a structured meal plan, with appropriate balanced meals and snacks to meet her nutritional needs. This meal plan will be more successful if it is a collaborative effort between the patient and the dietitian. This will serve to improve her nutritional status and reduce her preoccupation with thoughts of food as a result of starvation. It is preferable for the recovery process that the meal or snack be consumed in an area reserved for eating, for example the kitchen or dining room (Davis *et al.*, 1989). This will help to avoid having the urge to eat (which may lead to a binge) in other areas of the house. Once a meal or snack is completed, it is important for the person to remove herself from the kitchen or dining room. The act of brushing teeth immediately after a meal or snack may help to signal the end of the eating, and to prevent any desire for more food due to the taste of the toothpaste in her mouth.

A distraction of some sort is necessary after eating, in order to prevent worrying about the food just consumed. The person recovering from bulimia nervosa should be encouraged to call a friend, go for a walk, or engage in a mind-absorbing task.

Some individuals recovering from bulimia nervosa find it helpful to keep a log or journal to record events of the day and their feelings related to them. This may help the individual to discover what emotions may trigger a binge. This may also help her to know during which times of the day she may be more vulnerable.

Often, for a person with bulimia nervosa, eating is a very important source of pleasure. It is, therefore, very useful for her to make a list of other ways to experience pleasure that she may substitute for eating. This list may include such things as listening to favorite music, taking a bubble bath, going to a movie, etc.

Exercising is often done by the person suffering from bulimia nervosa as a way of burning calories. In fact, it may be seen by that person as an alternative method of purging. It is important to help her to change that mind-set, and learn to exercise for pleasure rather than to burn calories. One way of doing that is to encourage enjoyable 'activities', i.e. walking, cycling, rollerblading, swimming, etc., rather than the typical 'body-shaping' exercises such as crunches and jumping jacks. If the person recovering from bulimia has been regularly weighing herself, she should be encouraged to stop this practice. Focusing on healthy eating habits and healthy lifestyle rather than weight needs to be emphasized. Regular weighing will likely sabotage her efforts at normal eating without purging, due to her reaction to normal weight fluctuations.

Both the dietitian and the person recovering from bulimia must accept that this is a long, slow process, and that every step forward is positive. No one ever quits purging all at once. It has to be a gradual process that the individual adapts to physically and psychologically over a period of time.

# Weight maintenance and follow-up

Once the person recovering from an eating disorder has achieved her ideal weight, one of two things must happen. If she is an adolescent not yet finished her linear growth and development, she needs to continue to grow and gain weight normally. If she is an adult who has completed her linear growth and development, she needs to learn how to maintain her weight in a healthy range.

The process required to allow normal growth and weight gain, or to promote maintenance of ideal weight are one and the same. If nutritional needs for age and activity level are being met the body will maintain appropriate weight.

Despite having had many months of nutritional counseling in the process of achieving ideal weight, the individual recovering from an eating disorder is at risk of relapse and having difficulty in maintaining her weight in the ideal range. The dietitian should be prepared to provide follow-up support for periods of time that may range from several months to several years depending on the patient. Often, just knowing that she will have a check-in visit with the dietitian helps the individual to continue to maintain her healthy eating habits and her healthy weight. One young woman this dietitian worked with found it impossible to maintain her ideal weight until she was given repeated reassurances that she would not be abandoned by the dietitian if she was seen as being fully recovered, by being able to maintain her ideal weight.

Follow-up visits are a good time to assess not only current eating habits, and whether nutritional needs are being met, but also feelings about food and eating. In this way, it is to be hoped that problems can be caught at an early stage, and the individual can be helped to avoid becoming entrenched in eating disorder behaviors again.

The decision about discharge from nutritional counseling follow-up must be a joint one, between the recovered individual and the dietitian. Over time, it will become obvious to both at the follow-up visit that things are going well and the recovered individual truly has her life back. This is the appropriate time for discharge always with the understanding that if the person who has recovered from her eating disorder starts to experience difficulties in eating or with feelings about eating, she may come back for additional help from the dietitian.

# Medical management

*James A McSherry*

Effective community-based medical management of persons struggling with an eating disorder requires family physicians who have an interest in the affected person, some knowledge of eating disorders and their medical complications, access to specialized hospital-based services and a willingness to be part of a collaborative team of health professionals. Family physicians are usually called upon to monitor the affected person's physical health and to participate in the overall care plan to the extent appropriate given the prevailing circumstances, e.g. accessibility and affordability of counseling, nutritional and other services not provided by health insurance plans. Family physicians may be the most accessible health professionals in many communities and will likely be called upon to play an expanded role as therapist in that situation. An ability to understand the fears, beliefs and attitudes of affected persons and to translate that into 'common ground' acceptable to the individual patient and physician is fundamental to success as physician or as physician/therapist. Family physicians are perhaps uniquely qualified to help affected persons acknowledge the connections between their behaviors and their symptoms, observable physical problems and abnormal laboratory test results.

Information about family physicians' knowledge and practice behaviors with regard to eating disorders is scanty. One UK study (Hugo *et al.*, 2000) found that referral rates to a specialized eating-disorder service were higher in teaching group practices geographically close to the service, where there was at least one female physician. The physicians who had qualified in the UK, possessed a higher qualification in general/family practice and offered full contraceptive services. These characteristics identify a culture-specific cohort of younger family physicians whose training has increased their detection and referral rates. However, the study did not measure the extent to which practices offered treatment to their patients affected by eating disorders either before or instead of referral. It would be reasonable to assume that family physicians referred their most seriously affected patients for specialist attention, particularly since it has been recommended that recent onset binge eating and bulimia nervosa should be treated in general/family practice before referral (Royal College of Psychiatrists, 1992). A study of family physicians practising in a Canadian university city

(Boule and McSherry, 2000) found that respondents listed their top three educational needs about eating disorders as screening, diagnostic issues and management planning.

Publication of the Practice guideline for the treatment of patients with eating disorders (American Psychiatric Association, 2000) has provided clinicians with a useful source of evidence-based information and recommendations for treating eating disorders on lines that reflect current 'best practice'. The medical management of persons with eating disorders is not yet likely to be within the scope of everyday family practice. Nonetheless, the APA guideline offers information in sufficient detail that family physicians who follow its evidence-based recommendations should be able to diagnose eating disorders, assess and monitor affected persons medically, identify and manage many of the medical complications, perform at least a rudimentary psychiatric evaluation and develop a management plan.

# Choice of therapy

Persons with eating disorders commonly exhibit a range of behaviors and attitudes of varying severity that place them on an 'at-risk' continuum for anorexia nervosa and bulimia nervosa with the 'EDNOS' category likely covering the majority of persons struggling with eating disorders seen in generalist practice. Equally well, there is a wide range of management techniques and interventions that can be tailored to the individual situation. No 'one size fits all' approach is likely to be successful in each and every case, and management plans must take individual characteristics into account when interventions are selected and applied to specific patients.

# Treatment aims

# Anorexia nervosa

The aims of treatment for persons affected by anorexia nervosa (American Psychiatric Association, 2000) include:

- restoration of normal weight
- management of physical complications

- encouragement of patients to engage in a treatment plan that restores healthy eating patterns
- provision of appropriate education regarding healthy eating, both content and process
- correction of maladaptive thoughts, attitudes and behaviors that are central to the condition
- treatment of associated psychiatric conditions
- enlistment of family support and provision of family therapy where necessary
- prevention of relapse.

Normal weight has been restored when post-pubertal females ovulate and have a normal menstrual cycle, when males have normal hormone profiles and libido (sexual drive), and when children and adolescents resume normal physical growth and development.

Successful management of physical complications, described in Chapter 1 and summarized in Table 1.1, depends on their recognition, hence the importance of an initial medical assessment and periodic monitoring. Clinical examination should have a particular focus on the cardiovascular system and should include an ECG and blood tests for electrolyte measurement.

Helping affected individuals engage in therapy is one of the most challenging aspects of eating-disorders management. Patients in the early stages of anorexia nervosa often experience a sense of euphoria and are reluctant to accept that there is anything wrong with their attitudes and behaviors, never mind compelling reasons to change them. That usually changes as malnutrition takes its toll on energy levels, mood, social involvement, athletic performance, academic achievement and general well-being. However, despite the dawning of realization that all is not well, the thoughts, attitudes and behaviors that have contributed to development of the eating disorder are usually now autonomous habits, difficult to break. The focus of management necessarily shifts to the correction of central thoughts, beliefs and attitudes that perpetuate problematic behaviors, e.g. when persons struggling with eating disorders make themselves vomit after meals in the mistaken belief that abdominal discomfort and distension after eating is related to immediate conversion of food to fat.

Re-education about diet, nutrition and healthy eating patterns usually requires the active participation of a nutritionist or therapeutic dietician as an essential team member. Eating disorders are not solely about nutrition, yet malnutrition may be the most immediate problem. Patients struggling with eating disorders can benefit substantially from a nutritionist's advice on correcting nutritional deficiencies, improving food choices and developing acceptable alternative eating plans that maximize the nutritional content of a diet that is usually restricted in both quality and quantity. Additionally, nutritionists who are knowledgeable about eating disorders can provide valuable coaching to patients struggling with anorexia, helping them to understand the normal physical experiences of hunger and satiety, experiences that affected persons have been deliberately suppressing for so long that they cannot now recognize them for what they are.

Persons affected by anorexia nervosa often experience marked anxiety around food and eating, together with symptoms of depression such as apathy, sleep disturbance, low self-esteem and social withdrawal (Halmi et al., 1991). The anxiety around food often extends to the social occasions where eating is customary and contributes to the social withdrawal normally associated with depression. Depression in anorexia nervosa is directly related to poor nutritional status (Cooper, 1995) and can only be treated effectively by improved nutrition and weight restoration. Antidepressant medications are usually reserved for persons affected by anorexia nervosa who display marked anxiety and persistent depression or obsessive–compulsive symptoms (American Psychiatric Association, 2000). Their use in anorexia nervosa tends to be less effective than in normal weight-depressed persons, produces more side effects and may be associated with an increased risk of serious medical complications. Tricyclic antidepressants like imipramine and amitriptyline may increase the risk of cardiac conduction abnormalities in patients who are purging and/or using laxatives. They are best avoided in underweight patients and those at risk of suicide (American Psychiatric Association, 2000). There is a risk of seizures associated with use of bupropion in patients who purge (Horne et al., 1988). Selective serotonin reuptake inhibitors (SSRIs) are an attractive option because of their relative freedom from side effects and low toxicity if taken in overdose, either by accident or design. However, experience with fluoxetine (Prozac) in depressed persons of normal weight has found that appetite reduction and weight loss are relatively common side effects, at least in the first months of treatment, thus limiting its use in underweight patients struggling with anorexia nervosa. The golden rule is that if antidepressants are strongly indicated in a particular patient, it is best to use small doses initially and to watch carefully for side effects.

The situation is different in weight-restored patients after discharge from hospital when the psychological sequelae of starvation are resolved or are resolving. One study (Kaye et al., 1991) found that fluoxetine use at that point was generally helpful, fluoxetine-treated patients (average dose 40 mg daily) having fewer rehospitalizations, less weight loss and fewer symptoms of depression than in non-treated patients.

# Bulimia nervosa

The goals (American Psychiatric Association, 2000) of bulimia therapy include:

- reducing the frequency and severity of binge eating and purging
- avoiding periods of food restriction

- improving problematic attitudes and behaviors regarding food, eating and weight
- treating associated conditions
- encouraging healthy exercise patterns
- dealing with underlying issues.

Persons affected by bulimia nervosa and bulimia-like behaviors need to establish a regular pattern of non-binge 'healthy' meals with attention to stabilizing calorie intake, expanding the range of food choices and avoiding food-intake restriction. This frequently means eating more to eat less, as problem eating behaviors are often mutually reinforcing. A reduction in the frequency and severity of eating binges will reduce the frequency and severity of purging behaviors, but is, in turn, dependent upon reductions in the frequency and length of periods of food restriction. The common pattern is one of periods of starvation that alternate with binge/purge cycles. Weight loss, at least in the mind of the affected person, is best achieved by stringent calorie reduction, but periods of stringent calorie reduction usually end in eating binges that produce overall weight gain because of the large amount of calories consumed and associated fluid retention. Many persons with bulimia nervosa experience weight fluctuations, and may maintain several wardrobes to match.

Co-morbid conditions are relatively common in women who struggle with syndromal variants of bulimia nervosa, i.e. conditions that are clearly clinically significant, but, while failing to meet strict diagnostic criteria, are frequently referred to as bulimia nervosa for simplicity's sake. About 35% of women with bulimia nervosa have problems with substance abuse (Halmi et al., 1991; Herzog et al., 1992). Others suffer from mood disorders, mainly anxiety and depression, and PTSDs related to mental, physical and sexual abuse.

Effective treatment plans for persons struggling with bulimia nervosa usually include appropriate combinations of nutrition counseling, cognitive-behavioral therapy, individual psychotherapy, group therapy, family and marital therapy and medical therapy. Nutrition counseling corrects misinformation and helps construct healthy eating plans, cognitive-behavioral therapy links symptoms and behaviors to attitudes and beliefs, while individual psychotherapy provides person-specific insights into the origins of contributory attitudes and beliefs. Group therapy provides peer feedback and support, family and marital therapy address aspects of relationships and medical therapy treats associated mood disorders and medical complications.

Antidepressants certainly improve symptoms of anxiety and depression in persons affected by bulimia nervosa, but have the additional benefit of reducing the frequency of bingeing and purging even in non-depressed persons. Tricyclic antidepressants like imipramine (Pope et al., 1983), desipramine (Hughes et al., 1986) and amitriptyline (Mitchell and Groat, 1984) have been proven useful in randomized controlled trials, but their acceptability is limited by their potential for side effects like dry mouth, constipation, sedation and weight gain, and the risk of inducing cardiac conduction abnormalities in persons who have low potassium levels or who may attempt suicide by overdose of prescribed medications. The antidepressant bupropion is not recommended for use in bulimic patients who purge, because of the risk of inducing seizures. Monoamine oxidase inhibitor (MAOI) antidepressant drugs are contraindicated in the management of bulimia (American Psychiatric Association, 2000) because of the uncontrolled eating and probability of reaction when tyramine-containing foods are ingested. The only medication currently approved by the US Food and Drug Administration for use in bulimia nervosa is the selective serotonin reuptake inhibitor (SSRI) fluoxetine, although others, notably fluvoxamine, are currently being studied.

Curiously, while researchers find that cognitive-behavioral therapy is more effective than pharmacotherapy, experienced clinicians tend to favor pharmacotherapy (drug treatment) and the likelihood is that the cognitive-behavioral therapy provided to research-study participants is either qualitatively or quantitatively different from that available in routine practice. The combination of pharmacotherapy with cognitive-behavioral therapy tends to produce results that are superior to either treatment alone (American Psychiatric Association, 2000).

# The care plan

Making the diagnosis is one thing, determining the best treatment for the individual affected by an eating disorder is something else entirely. Choices of treatment setting generally lie between treatment in the community with medical monitoring, admission to a general medical unit, admission to a psychiatric unit or admission to a specialized eating-disorders residential or day-hospital program. Some individuals may have an experience of all these settings in the course of their struggle. There is evidence that persons with severe eating disorders or their complications do better in specialized inpatient units than in general psychiatry or medical units. Indeed, in the author's experience, patients admitted to general psychiatry units typically have their medical needs neglected, while those admitted to medical units have their mental health needs ignored. The main factors that determine the most appropriate site or setting for care (American Psychiatric Association, 2000; Fichter, 1995) are weight, cardiac status and presence or absence of metabolic abnormalities. They include:

- presence or absence of medical complications, e.g. vomiting blood, low potassium, abnormal vital signs, etc.

- potential for suicide
- weight as a percentage of healthy body weight (for adults)
- rate of weight loss (for children)
- motivation to recover and ability to co-operate
- presence or absence of co-morbid disorders like substance abuse, depression and anxiety
- degree of structure and supervision required
- potential for self-care and ability to control exercise
- frequency and severity of purging behaviors
- adequacy of social supports and relationships
- living situation and proximity to treatment resources.

Someone who has suicidal intent or a plan, an adult whose weight is below 75% of normal healthy weight for age and height and a child whose food refusal is causing rapid weight loss should generally be admitted to hospital. An adult whose pulse rate is 40 beats per minute or less, whose blood pressure is less than 90/60 mm mercury, whose body temperature is lower that 97.0°F, who is dehydrated and/or has an electrolyte imbalance and/or a low potassium level should generally be admitted to hospital. An adult with evidence of cardiac, liver or kidney abnormalities should be admitted to hospital.

Lack of motivation to recover, poor co-operation with treatment in anything other than a highly structured environment, need for supervision to prevent compulsive exercising, and need for tube feeding or supervision during and after meals all strongly indicate the desirability of hospital admission. Concurrent substance abuse generally requires treatment in a residential setting. Additional factors indicating a need for treatment in a residential setting include living too far from a treatment center, to live at home while participating in an outpatient program, living alone without adequate social supports and severe family problems that prejudice structured management plans at home.

On the other hand, persons struggling with eating disorders can generally be managed safely in a community setting if:

- they are medically stable and do not require tube feeding, intravenous fluids or daily laboratory tests
- they have no suicidal intent or plan
- they are over 85% of normal healthy weight for age and height
- they have some degree of insight and are willing to co-operate
- they do not abuse alcohol or drugs
- they are able to control their complusion to exercise
- they can reduce the frequency and severity of purging behaviors in a non-structured setting
- they have supportive social and emotional relationships and
- they live near the treatment setting.

# Refeeding phenomena

Even when persons struggling with an eating disorder move from a restricting phase to one of refeeding in response to treatment, the medical problems are not over. Refeeding may be associated with:

- depression, fatigue and lassitude as endorphin production falls
- abdominal fullness and discomfort, bloating and cramps due to delayed stomach emptying and increased food bulk
- rapid weight gain when purging behaviors are stopped
- blood electrolyte abnormalities when dehydration is corrected, e.g. low calcium and potassium
- edema due to massive fluid retention possibly progressing to congestive cardiac failure
- acute dilatation or perforation of the stomach, particularly if nasogastric tube feeding has been instituted
- repeat puberty with acne, menstrual cramps, breast development as normal endocrine function is gradually restored.

Some of these phenomena are likely to be temporary and of nuisance value only, e.g. abdominal bloating and discomfort after eating, and rapid weight gain when purging behaviors cease. However, if patients have not been made aware that these things are likely to happen, then their occurrence has the potential for being misinterpreted in accordance with the belief system of the individual patient. Rapid weight gain may cause great alarm as an affected person becomes anxious that weight increase will continue indefinitely at the same rate, reinforcing fears of fatness and triggering a return to restricting or purging behaviors. Abdominal bloating may be interpreted as instant conversion of ingested food to fat with a similar return to problematic behaviors. Repeat puberty comes after significant amounts of weight have been regained. It may reinforce previous misgivings about changing bodily shape and fears of fatness with resulting relapse unless patients are carefully prepared about what to expect with refeeding.

Other phenomena are serious, potentially life-threatening and require urgent medical intervention, e.g. congestive cardiac failure (shortness of breath, generalized edema, abnormal physical findings in heart and lungs), acute gastric dilatation and perforation. Fortunately, they are unlikely to happen except in the institutional setting when severely malnourished individuals are treated by nasogastric tube feeding or parenteral nutrition.

If fluid retention is a major problem and weakens an individual patient's commitment to healing, then potassium sparing diuretics, e.g. spironolactone, are a safe and effective drug therapy (Goldbloom and Kennedy, 1995). Abdominal bloating can be treated effectively using prokinetic drugs (domperidone, etc.)

before meals (American Psychiatric Association, 2000) and GERD can be managed using antisecretory drugs (H2 blockers, proton pump inhibitors) and prokinetic drugs before meals and before bed.

# Common ground

The key concepts of finding common ground are: defining the problems, the goals and the respective roles of physician and patient (Brown *et al.*, 1995).

The process of finding common ground is essentially one of exploration, reconciling the patient's fears, attitudes and behaviors with the physician's concerns and treatment strategies. The following case study is instructive.

### Case study
Michelle, a 17-year-old female, presented to a physician for routine monitoring of anorexia nervosa of bulimic subtype. Her parents were divorcing and the situation had become particularly unpleasant in the previous week as each parent sought to enlist support from Michelle and her two brothers. She had lost 1 kg in the week since her last visit and admitted that the frequency of her self-induced vomiting had increased from once most days to twice every day. Additionally, she reported an increasing and formerly uncharacteristic preoccupation with cleaning and tidying. Her pulse rate (64) and blood pressure (90/60 mm Hg with no significant postural drop) were unchanged from the previous visit, but her potassium level had dropped to 2.8 meq/l from 3.6 meq/l a week earlier.

The physician explained that the weight loss, more-frequent vomiting and low potassium level were of major concern, particularly in association with obsessive–compulsive cleaning rituals. The question of hospitalization was brought up, given the highly problematic home situation, but Michelle begged to be allowed to continue at school because of imminent examinations, the support she was getting from her friends and a feeling that she was being punished for other people's problems.

When asked how she could reduce her energy expenditure and increase her energy intake, Michelle volunteered to eliminate her gym workout sessions (three sessions per week, each of one and a half hours' duration) for a week, to try hard to reduce the frequency of her vomiting from twice every day to no more than once a day, and to take daily potassium supplements. The physician agreed that this was a workable plan. Michelle gave a commitment to do her best to make it happen on the understanding that hospital admission remained an option. At her next visit a week later Michelle had regained the lost kg, her blood pressure was 110/70 and her potassium level 3.2.

In this situation, two divergent perspectives of the same situation were brought together in a management strategy that was realistic and recognized the over-riding imperatives of both parties. The emphasis was on jointly discovering common ground. The physician knew that he had compulsory legal powers at his disposal, but offered voluntary admission as a means of drawing Michelle's attention to the gravity of her situation and the destructive effect of the current home environment. Michelle's response was one of self-assertion, to point out that she had strongly supportive peer relationships that sustained her, to emphasize her need for personal autonomy in a world that had lost its previously valid reference points and to stress the importance of her academic achievements. Michelle recognized the importance and relevance of her physician's advice. Her physician saw her need for control in some areas of her life.

# Subsequent medical monitoring

Medical monitoring, the ongoing observation of the affected person's condition and response to changes, should focus on:

- the abnormalities found at the initial medical examination
- the known medical consequences of the individual patient's behavior
- new symptoms or signs
- the patient's mood, including risk of suicide
- usefulness of or indications for medical therapies, including antidepressant drugs

Generally speaking, this will include:

- checking weight, blood pressure and general cardiac status
- taking blood for electrolyte measurement
- assessing progress/severity of abnormalities found at previous examinations
- performing an ECG – not necessarily indicated at each visit.

Persons with eating disorders are often reluctant to be weighed in the doctor's office even though weight is an important piece of the malnourished, underweight patient's medical evaluation. It is usually possible to negotiate an acceptable compromise such as weighing every other visit or weighing while the patient faces away from the scales and given a verdict regarding general progress. The doctor's need for information and the patient's fear of the scales are not necessarily irreconcilable. Many persons affected by anorexia nervosa will readily resort to strategies that temporarily increase weight, e.g. drinking large volumes of water immediately before weighing in, concealing bunches of keys and quantities of loose change in their pockets, fasting rigorously until the day before a doctor's appointment and then binge eating to retain fluid, etc. Patients may have to be weighed in an examination gown and have their urine tested for specific gravity to detect spurious weight maintenance or gain.

Frequencies of visits and intervals between them depend on the individual patient's condition and whether or not other care providers are actively involved in the patient's management plan. The patient whose purging behavior is so frequent and severe that daily electrolyte checks are required should be admitted to a specialized eating-disorders unit, or at least hospitalized. For most patients, a weekly medical visit should be adequate and the interval between visits can be lengthened when patients are medically stable.

Optimal management of the person affected by an eating disorder requires the active involvement of a collaborative, interdisciplinary team whose members may well include, but not necessarily be limited to, a psychiatrist, a clinical psychologist, a family physician, a medical specialist, a dentist, a social worker, a nutritionist, a family therapist, a personal counselor or other individual whose advice is respected by the affected person. Not everyone will always be the 'ball-carrier', but each may be called upon to contribute their personal talents and professional skills to the care plan.

While this kind of team, formally constructed, is usually only available within specialized centers offering residential or day-hospital programs, community-based health professionals can and do organize themselves into informal multi-disciplinary networks where shared care is possible and efficacious. Caregiver gender and cultural differences may limit the contribution an individual team member can make to the care of individual patients.

Communication between health professionals is the major problem in this 'virtual' program. Each member must take care to acquire permission in advance for communication with other members of the network regarding persons with eating disorders who are receiving care in this community-based model.

# Rose's story

Being in recovery now offers an interesting perspective on what was and wasn't helpful to me during my battle with an eating disorder. My personal view is that being in recovery doesn't mean that I'm cured. I still struggle with thoughts of wanting to lose weight. I still have a distorted image of myself, and I still have to work on quieting my EDV. I hope that one day I won't feel the way I do. I hope that one day, when I sit down to a meal, I won't have that momentary thought of 'Oh my God, why am I eating this, it has so many calories.' Perhaps that will come with time. Yet I wonder. My eating disorder has been such a big part of my life (at times it was my life) that maybe this is as good as it gets. Perhaps I will have to continue to battle this everyday for the rest of my life. I hope not. I hope with continued therapy I can one day be truly free from my eating disorder.

The things that I found most helpful leading up to and during my recovery were as follows. I must state here that no one thing was more helpful than any other; rather, they worked together to bring me to the place I am now. Therefore these are in no particular order.

# Antidepressant medication

In order to begin working on the precursors to my eating disorder it was necessary to bring my depression to a level where I wasn't suicidal, and at a reasonably healthy mental functioning point. It took quite a while to find the right combination of medications that worked for me. Some medications would work for a while and then suddenly stop working. With others the side effects were too harsh. My doctor and I experimented with many types of medications and dosages until we finally found the combination that has worked for me for the past four years.

# Therapy

Two or three times a week at my worst, now I go twice a week. Since I didn't see that I came from a dysfunctional family, and disassociated myself from traumas in my life, I had no comprehension of myself. I didn't see the connection between my life and my eating disorder. I accepted my family's problems as my own, and blamed myself for the dysfunction. I didn't realize that I was a perfectionist. I though all people lived the way I did. I was convinced that I was a monster of a human being. Therapy allowed me to see the distortion of my thought processes and how they allowed the perpetuation of self-destruction and self-loathing.

# Support group

Once out of the treatment center, it was necessary for me to find support with people who understood what I had gone through and what I was going through. I was also able to share experiences with others and help them. This made me feel valuable and helped my self-esteem. The support group was particularly helpful when I found myself sliding backwards. Since there were people there in various stages of recovery, talking to those who had stopped a slide was more effective than talking to my doctor.

# My family doctor

I would see my family doctor once a week. For blood tests, to monitor my weight and to chat about how my eating was going. It was helpful to check in with my doctor to keep focused on getting healthier physically. The weigh-ins were the most difficult because they kept me focused on the numbers.

I stopped weighing myself at home, and found this to be helpful. I discussed this with my doctor and she started weighing me with my back to the scale and not telling me the numbers, just if I was up or down, but not by how much. With this, I broke the numbers obsession. I no longer know how much I weigh. I don't want to know. I just want to know that my weight is okay.

Several treatment approaches were not helpful. My family doctor was unfamiliar with the intricacies of eating disorder management at the time of my diagnosis. Because of this it was very easy for me to maintain my eating-disorder and lead her to think that I had the intent of wanting help. I would see her once a week. She would say she wanted to see me, so I would make the appointment. My husband was happy because he thought I was getting help. I was maintaining my eating disorder all the while. I would put weights in my pockets so that I could manipulate my weight and make it appear as though I was maintaining my weight, while continuing to loose weight. As my disorder continued she knew that I was getting weaker and sicker. She knew that something was not right and I needed hospitalization.

My experiences with my hospitalizations were both positive and negative. If intense therapy could have been provided to me in combination with medical/nutritional management I feel that these two treatment approaches would have been more successful.

# Taking control

I now am able to manage my eating disorder. It was a long and hard road; I am in what is known as recovery. Some of the ways in which I manage my eating disorder are as follows. I do not weigh myself. My husband or my doctor weighs me. They do not tell me what the number is, just if I've gone up or down. Although at times it's incredibly hard not to try and turn around and see the number on the scale, I stop myself. I have no idea what the number is. I know that if I were to see the number I would relapse. I know the number is in three digits, and that is hard for me to handle. Actually seeing the number would make me want to get it back down to a two-digit number and the whole cycle would start again. One day I decided that I wasn't going to weigh myself anymore. It was one of the most difficult decisions in my recovery. Every morning the scale would call to me, and everyday I would resist. As time passed it became easier. This I think was the first and major step I took to take control of my own recovery. I knew I had to get away from the numbers, and this was the way to do it. In fact, I try to stay away from any number-oriented activity such as looking at calories on food packaging and ordering the lowest-calorie item on the menu; most of all trying to catch myself when I begin to calculate calories consumed.

This leads me to another important step in my recovery. I try to be aware of any thoughts or patterns that are related to disordered eating. If I stop eating a certain food and say to myself that I suddenly don't like it, and it happens to be a high-calorie food, I question the motives behind the sudden dislike. I am aware of thoughts contributing to eating-disorder patterns. I can identify my EDV and talk back to it. Most importantly I know that my eating disorder has nothing to do with food. If I start to exhibit signs of reoccurrence I discuss this with my therapist and try to discover the cause. I am aware of triggers for me. Being able to identify these helps me to catch a slide before it gets out of my control. Some of my personal triggers are as follows: stressful situations (whether they relate to work or family situations), periods of depression, quick weight gain due to an illness, overexposure to fashion magazines at vulnerable times or being in constant contact with someone who is very thin. Being around a group of people who are constantly dieting as well as trying on clothes from last season that no longer fit me leads me to focus on my own weight gain and eating. The most difficult thing for me is being in close constant contact with a friend who is still in the midst of an eating disorder. This makes me want to start restricting and old thought patterns return quickly.

My long battle with an eating disorder has taken its toll on my body. I have a heart complication consisting of arrhythmias, particularly tachycardia, for which I need to take medication. Bouts of hypokalemia are also controlled with medication. I have osteoporosis. I am 36 years old and have the bone density of a woman in her mid 70s. I have bowel problems resulting from many years of laxative abuse. My hair has thinned and both my skin and body have aged prematurely. The growth of lanugo on various parts of my body has not gone away. I have thyroid problems as well. These illnesses are all directly relating to my eating disorder.

# Family and friends

I'm often asked what can one do or say to help a loved one with an eating disorder. How should they act? First you must remember that all people are individuals, and what works for one person may not necessarily work for another, but there are common threads. These are my observations and experiences through coping with my own illness.

The first and most important point is this; do not assume to know how the person feels. Unless you've suffered from an eating disorder yourself, **You don't.** Do not say the words 'I know how you feel'. **You don't.** Do not say, 'I have days when I feel fat, too'. During an eating disorder those words take on a whole new meaning. It doesn't have anything to do with weight; the individual could be 70 lbs when they say 'I feel fat'. Do not say, 'I've had down days too, and this is how I made myself feel better'. Depression is a serious illness that often accompanies an eating disorder. Depression is not a 'down day'. Unless you are a trained professional, do not assume to know the way the mind works in the midst of depression. Do not be critical. Do not put the person down. It does not matter if you're having a bad day, and it slips out. This is very detrimental. Even if you think that you're not being critical, it may seem that way to the individual. They could take it that way, feeling worse about themselves and withdrawing. If you are having conflicts in your family due to a member having an eating disorder, try not to argue in front of them. If you need to talk about the family member or vent your frustrations, do not let the individual hear you. You may be frustrated and feel as though you are cushioning them. Without this they may feel that they are causing even more pain to the ones they love. They may blame themselves and become even more entrenched in their eating disorder.

Try and remove as many pressures of everyday life as possible. No matter what they say, or do, love them. Try to be as unselfish as possible. Your academic and financial expectations are not important at this point. What is important is that the individual knows that you love them unconditionally. We are perfectionists, and put enough pressure on ourselves. The last thing we need is to feel additional pressure from family and friends. All you can do is make it as easy and comfortable as possible for the individual to get better.

Understand that nothing you can say or do will make the eating disorder go away. If you ask, 'How are you?', be prepared to listen; really listening and not interrupt. Again, don't try to understand. It won't make sense. It's called an eating disorder because it's disordered, and so is the thinking. If they should get angry and say hurtful things, understand it has little to do with you. This is unconditional love. An eating disorder has nothing to do with food, it's an emotional state. We feel broken inside. If we appear happy, we are probably pretending. We are masters of emotional camouflage. It's probably because we've lost weight, or happen to be having a good day. It's not because we're cured. So don't feel let down if the next day it's 'back to normal'. This is not necessarily your fault. A therapist can help you with your own emotions and frustrations. You can't rely on the individual to get you through this. They simply can't help you deal with your issues surrounding their eating disorder. They're having enough trouble getting from day to day.

Don't try to be an expert on eating disorders by giving advice and examples of other sufferers' successes. This will only serve to make the individual feel inferior and more of a failure. Educate yourself as much as possible, but understand that unless you've been there, you will never know how we feel or what we are going through.

Do not make comments surrounding food or eating. If they are not eating, comments surrounding that fact or your displeasure with it will only serve to reaffirm their convictions. On the other hand, do not comment if they are eating or making an attempt to eat regardless of whether you are simply joyous to see them eating or just trying to be supportive. We are very aware of the fact that we are eating, and do not need anyone to bring it to our attention and make us feel self-conscious of the fact. Starting to eat again is a very difficult task for us, and one that we need to do for ourselves, not for anyone else.

Do not use the word 'thin'. It is a word associated with success. You can tell them that they are extremely emaciated. We don't see ourselves the way others do, we have a distorted image of ourselves. Once the individual begins to gain weight, commenting or complementing them on this is a very tricky road. Depending on the individual, this one comment could cause a relapse. The individual is very aware of the slightest gain in weight, and probably very uncomfortable with that fact. They will also probably torment you with the question 'Do I look fat?' This may seem like a ridiculous and insignificant question to you, but is very serious to the individual. Tell them the truth. They won't believe you, but your comment will stick in their mind. Most of all ... love them, no matter what, without exceptions.

I understand that it is difficult for family members and friends to watch someone they love going through an eating disorder. But you must understand that it is much more difficult for the individual.

When I asked my husband what it was that he did to help me get through my eating disorder, he answered, 'I worked hard at doing nothing.' At first I didn't understand what he meant. After some thought I realized that he meant that he tried to keep things as normal in our household as possible.

Looking back now, I see some of the compromises and selfless behavior on his part. He took over the day-to-day management of our household. Not only was this a goodwill gesture on his part, but eventually a necessary one. I was not capable of managing even the smallest details. My day was consumed with thoughts surrounding food and dealing with my depression.

He figured out that if he asked me what I had eaten during the day, I would lie to him. I would leave empty containers of food, or dirtied plates for him to see, thinking I was fooling him, all the while losing weight. It didn't take him long to discover that I was throwing out the food and just smearing the plates with food. He learned that it was useless to interrogate me about my daily food intake or about food in general.

He didn't put any pressure on me regarding my declining weight. The only thing he did insist on was that I keep seeing my therapist and my family doctor. He put his trust in them. Somehow he knew that it was up to me to decide whether I wanted to get better, and nothing he could say would change that.

I'm not trying to suggest that all was perfect in our world. It wasn't. We both went through our own personal hell. We learned together through our own and each other's mistakes.

Without him I couldn't have gotten through this. If it weren't for his unconditional love and support, I wouldn't be here to write this.

# Conclusion

This chapter provides a detailed summary of the work of four key health professionals who specialize in the treatment of persons with eating disorders. The fifth contributor is the patient Rose, whose voice provides a first-person account of the experience of living with an eating disorder. Her story is realistic, informative, heartfelt and profoundly moving. Her contribution adds an essential component to a patient-centered treatment plan, and reminds the reader that this disorder (anorexia nervosa) has a very human form. It also shows how deeply affected other family members are by the presence of an eating-disordered person in the family. The integration of the experience of the client, combined with the expertise of the professionals, provides a fuller account of the course of the illness and its management. Patient-centered care is a commitment to an ideal, as well as a respectful approach to medical practice. It ensures that the patient's voice is heard loud and clear, and that the process of assessment and treatment is truly a collaborative one.

Patient-centered care invites a unique partnership between clinician and patient. In the case of persons with eating disorders the establishment of a therapeutic alliance may take some time, and requires additional patience and tact on behalf of the clinician.

It encourages collaboration in the discovery (diagnostic) process. Though the disorder may be quite visible to the clinician (as in the case of anorexia nervosa) it is unwise to assume that the client has also perceived the problem and arrived at the same conclusion, i.e. a diagnosis of an eating disorder and a commitment to further investigation and treatment. Frequently this is a difficult diagnosis for patients to accept. Despite 'acceptance' at one level, there is often marked resistance at another level to the realities of this disorder. For the clinician, care must be taken in not jumping to conclusions before adequate medical investigations have been completed.

The following summarizes the key components of patient-centered care in treating eating disorders.

- It means listening carefully to the voice of the client, and privileging their experience in the therapeutic process.
- It implies a respect for the patient's rights to be fully informed.
- It acknowledges the patient's rights in all decision making processes.
- It attempts to demystify the process by encouraging mutual understanding of complex issues.
- It is commitment to the use of a common language of care, respect and compassion.
- It makes the clinician more transparent and less distant from the client.
- It promotes a more equal relationship and lessens professional hierarchy.
- It minimizes power and control issues which are especially important in understanding and treating persons with eating disorders.

In conclusion, establishing common ground builds on the notion of the importance of the therapeutic alliance between patient and team. The critical aspect of integration and co-ordination of psychological, familial, nutritional and medical aspects of care cannot be overemphasized. Without effective communication between clinicians, and a high degree of interdisciplinary co-ordination, the very real possibility exists of poor management and wasted time and effort by all concerned. On the other hand, the outlook for people with eating disorders and their families is immeasurably improved by solid team work and good patient-centered care.

# References

American Psychiatric Association (2000) Practice guidelines for the treatment of patients with eating disorders (revision). *Am J Psychiatry.* **157** (Supplement): 1–39.

Anderson H and Goolishan H (1988) Human systems as linguistic systems: preliminary and evolving ideas about the implications for clinical theory. *Fam Process.* **27**(4): 371–93.

Beaumont PJV, Beaumont CC, Touyz SW and Williams H (1997) Nutritional counseling and supervised exercise. In: DM Garner and RE Garfinkel (eds) *Handbook of Treatment for Eating Disorders.* Guilford Press, New York.

Berg FM (1996) Dysfunctional eating: a new concept. *Healthy Weight J.* **10**(5): 88–92.

Boule C and McSherry JA (2000) *Family physicians' knowledge, attitudes and beliefs about eating disorders.* Trillium Primary Care Research Forum, McMaster University, Canada.

Brown C (1993) Feminist therapy: power, ethics and control. In: C Brown and K Jasper (eds) *Consuming Passions: feminist approaches to weight preoccupation and eating disorders.* Second Story Press, Toronto, Canada.

Brown JB, Weston WW and Stewart M (1995) Finding common ground. In: M Stewart, JB Brown, WW Weston *et al.* (eds) *Patient-Centered Medicine: transforming the clinical method*. Sage Publications, Thousand Oaks, CA.

Cooper Z (1995) Development and maintenance of eating disorders. In: KD Brownell and CG Fairburn (eds) *Eating Disorders and Obesity: a comprehensive handbook*. Guilford Press, New York.

Crisp AH (1997) Anorexia nervosa as flight from growth: assessment and treatment based on the model. In: DM Garner and PE Garfinkel (eds) *Handbook of Treatment for Eating Disorders*. Guilford Press, New York.

Dare C and Eisler I (1997) Family therapy for anorexia nervosa. In: DN Garner and PE Garfinkel (eds) *Handbook of Treatment for Eating Disorders*. Guilford Press, New York.

Dare C, Eisler I, Russell GF and Szmukier GL (1990) The clinical and theoretical impact of trial of family therapy in anorexia nervosa. *J Marital Fam Ther*. **16**: 39–57.

Davis R, Dearing S, Faulkner J *et al.* (1989) *The Road to Recovery: a manual for participants in the psychoeducation group for bulimia nervosa*. The Toronto Hospital, Toronto General Division, Toronto, ON, Canada.

de Shazer S (1982) *Patterns of Brief Family: an ecosystemic approach*. Guilford Press, New York.

Eisler I, Dare C, Russell GF *et al.* (1997) Family and individual therapy in anorexia nervosa: a five-year follow-up. *Arch Gen Psychiatry*. **54**: 1025–30.

Fairburn CG (1997) Interpersonal psychotherapy for bulimia nervosa. In: DM Garner and PE Garfinkel (eds) *Handbook of Treatment for Eating Disorders*. Guilford Press, New York.

Fichter MM (1995) Inpatient treatment of anorexia nervosa. In: KE Brownell and CG Fairburn (eds) *Eating Disorders and Obesity: a comprehensive handbook*. Guilford Press, New York.

Garner DM (1997) Psychoeducational principles in treatment. In: DM Garner and PE Garfinkel (eds) *Handbook of Treatment for Eating Disorders*. Guilford Press, New York.

Garner DM, Vitousek KM and Pike KM (1997) Cognitive–behavioral therapy for anorexia nervosa. In: DM Garner and PE Garfinkel (eds) *Handbook of Treatment for Eating Disorders*. Guilford Press, New York.

Goldbloom DS and Kennedy SH (1995) Medical complications of anorexia nervosa. In: KD Brownell and GG Fairburn (eds) *Eating Disorders and Obesity: a comprehensive handbook*. Guilford Press, New York.

Goodsitt A (1997) Eating disorders: a self-psychological perspective. In: DM Garner and PE Garfinkel (eds) *Handbook of Treatment for Eating Disorders* (2e). Guilford Press, New York.

Hall L and Cohn L (1999) *Bulimia: a guide to recovery*. Gurze Books, Carlsbad, CA.

Halmi KA, Eckert E, Marchi P *et al.* (1991) Co-morbidity of psychiatric diagnoses in anorexia nervosa. *Arch Gen. Psychiatry*. **48**: 712–18.

Herzog DB, Keller MB, Sacks NR, Yeh CJ and Lavori PW (1992) Psychiatric co-morbidity in treatment-seeking anorexics and bulimics. *J Am Acad Child Adolesc Psychiatry*. **31**: 818–19.

Horne RL, Ferguson JM, Pope HJ *et al.* (1988) Treatment of bulimia with bupropion; A multi-center-controlled trial. *J Clin Psychiatry.* **49**: 262–6.

Howard CE and Krug Porzelius L (1999) The role of dieting in binge eating disorder: etiology and treatment implications. *Clin Psychol Rev.* **19**(1): 25–44.

Hsu LKG, Holben B and West S (1992) Nutritional counseling in bulimia nervosa. *Int J Eat Disord.* **11**(1): 55–62.

Hughes PL, Wells LA, Cunningham CJ and Ilstrup DM (1986) Treating bulimia with desipramine: a double-blind, placebo-controlled study. *Arch Gen Psychiatry.* **43**: 182–6.

Hugo P, Kendrick T, Reid F and Lacey H (2000) GP referral to an eating disorder service; why the wide variation. *Br J Gen Pract.* **50**: 380–3.

Hutchinson MG (1994) Imagining ourselves whole: a feminist approach to treating body image disorders. In: P Fallon, MA Katzman and SC Wooley (eds) *Feminist Perspectives on Eating Disorders.* Guilford Press, New York.

Kahn A (1994) Recovery through nutritional counseling. In: BP Kinoy (ed.) *Eating Disorders: new directions in treatment and recovery.* Columbia University Press, New York.

Kaplan AS and Olmsted MP (1997) Partial hospitalization. In: DM Garner and PE Garfinkel (eds) *Handbook of Treatment for Eating Disorders.* Guilford Press, New York.

Kaye WH, Weltzin TE, Hsu LK and Bulik CM (1991) Open trial of fluoxetine in patients with anorexia nervosa. *J Clin Psychiatry.* **52**: 464–71.

Kearney-Cooke A and Striegel-Moore R (1997) The etiology and treatment of body image disturbance. In: DM Garner and PE Garfinkel (eds) *Handbook of Treatment for Eating Disorders.* Guilford Press, New York.

Le Grange D (1999) Family therapy for adolescent anorexia nervosa. *J Clin Psychol.* **55**: 727–39.

McKisack C and Waller G (1997) Factors influencing the outcome of group psychotherapy for bulimia nervosa. *Int J Eat Disord.* **22**: 1–13.

Minuchin S, Rosmon SL and Baker L (1978) *Psychosomatic Families.* Harvard University Press, Cambridge, MA.

Mitchell JE and Groat R (1984) A placebo-controlled, double-blind trial of amitryptyline in bulimia. *J Clin Psychopharmacol.* **41**: 186–93.

Polivy J and Federoff I (1997) Group psychotherapy. In: DM Garner and PE Garfinkel (eds) *Handbook of Treatment for Eating Disorders.* Guilford Press, New York.

Pope HG, Hudson JI, Jonas JM and Yurgelun-Todd D (1983) Bulimia treated with imipramine: a placebo-controlled, double-blind study. *Am J Psychiatry.* **140**: 554–8.

Reiff DW and Lampson Reiff KK (1992) Cognitive distortions concerning nutrition, food, weight and health. In: *Eating Disorders: nutrition therapy in the recovery process.* Aspen Publishers, Inc, Gathersburg, MD.

Rorty M, Yager J and Rossotto E (1993) Why and how do women recover from bulimia nervosa?: the subjective appraisals of forty women recovered for a year or more. *Int J Eat Disord.* **14**: 249–60.

Rosen JC (1996) Body-image assessment and treatment in controlled studies of eating disorders. *Int J Eat Disord*. **20**: 331–43.

Royal College of Psychiatrists (1992) *Eating Disorders*. Council Report CR14. Royal College of Psychiatrists, London, UK.

Shekter-Wolfson L and Woodside DB (1990) *A Day Hospital Group Treatment Program for Anorexia Nervosa and Bulimia*. Brunner/Mazel, New York.

Shekter-Wolfson L, Woodside DB and Lackstrom J (1997) Social work treatment of anorexia and bulimia: guidelines for practice. *Res Soc Work Pract*. **7**: 5–31.

Stewart M, Brown JB, Weston WW *et al.* (1995) *Patient-Centered Medicine: transforming the clinical method*. Sage Publications, Thousand Oaks, CA.

Tomm K (1987) Interventive interviewing: part II: reflexive questioning as a means to enable self-healing. *Fam Process*. **27**: 167–83.

Vitousek K and Watson S (1998) Enhancing motivation for change in treatment-resistant eating disorders. *Clin Psychol Rev*. **18**: 391–420.

White M and Epston D (1990) *Narrative Means to Therapeutic Ends*. Norton, New York.

Wilson GT (1991) The addiction model of eating disorders: a critical analysis. *Adv Behav Res Therapy*. **13**: 27–72.

# 7

# A patient-centered approach to eating disorders: summary

*Kathleen M Berg*

This book has described a patient-centered approach to understanding the development, maintenance and treatment of eating disorders. The patient-centered method (Stewart *et al.*, 1995) in healthcare focuses on the uniqueness of an individual's experiences and emphasizes the importance of recognizing the whole person in understanding medical and social/psychological concerns. Within this method, the inclusion of the patient's voice is paramount. Patient ideas, feelings, experiences and expectations are encouraged and honored. In addition, patient-centered care advocates a collaborative approach to treatment wherein goal setting, choice of intervention and monitoring of progress are based on mutual decision-making between the patient and the clinicians involved.

In applying the patient-centered approach to eating disorders, the authors have advocated a multidimensional model acknowledging the complexity and wide variability of eating disorders. Even within the broad diagnostic categories of anorexia nervosa, bulimia nervosa and atypical eating disorders, sizable subgroups differ significantly in terms of their etiologies, and their symptom presentation on physical, behavioral, cognitive, social and family dimensions. Additional variables include the vulnerability of these conditions to perpetuating factors in an individual's life, their response to treatments, and their long term ramifications in the terms of nutritional wellbeing, physical and mental health, and social and familial functioning.

An important component of the multidimensional view is the unique experiencing of the eating disorder by the patient herself. A fundamental premise of this view is that expertise regarding contributory factors in the development and maintenance of eating disorders and the efficacy of therapeutic interventions resides with both the patient and the clinician. Multiple case reports, qualitative studies and excerpts from personal memoirs have been presented to elucidate the heterogeneity of patients' ideas and opinions, emotional experiences, expectations of clinicians and experiences regarding the impact of the eating disorder on ability to function in their lives personally, socially and vocationally.

Rose's story in Chapter 4 is exemplary with regards to the importance of understanding the whole person in the treatment of eating disorders. Through her personal exposé, Rose has described the complex interaction of cultural, familial, traumatic and individual predisposing factors which contributed to the development of her eating disorder. Her story is an excellent example of how multifaceted and dynamic an eating disorder can be in terms of both its symptomatic presentation and its impact on the many aspects and developmental stages of one's life. In addition, Rose has alerted clinicians to factors in the patient–clinician relationship and in the treatment selection process which can be either curative or iatrogenic in their impact. The importance of fostering a collaborative approach to the management of an eating disorder is certainly attested to here. The individual patient is more than a case of anorexia nervosa or bulimia nervosa. She has a unique personal, cultural and familial history, individualized symptomatology, unique needs and idiosyncratic reactions to both her disorder and to the various treatment approaches offered.

Given the multifactorial nature of eating disorders, the authors have also espoused a multidisciplinary model for outpatient treatment. This team approach includes the shared expertise of the psychologist, the family therapist, the physician and the dietitian. To be effective, it must be collaborative and patient-focused. The clinician who undermines the contributions of other professions, who dismisses the patient's ideas, preferences and feelings or who ignores the impact of the eating disorder on the family adversely affects the healing process and seriously compromises the patient's chances for recovery.

Within the multidisciplinary approach to eating disorders, the focus is on an eclectic model and individual tailoring of treatment programs to meet the patient's needs. Common ground between patient and clinician is achieved through mutual goal setting, open communication and encouraging an interactive process throughout the treatment process including assessment, management and follow-up.

Finally, the efficacy of the patient-centered approach is rooted in the quality of the patient–clinician relationship. The clinician most effective in promoting the development of a therapeutic alliance is one who demonstrates a high level of self-awareness, and communicates several important attributes including empathic understanding, warmth, respect, patience, flexibility and genuineness.

Cutbacks to healthcare have resulted in increased stress on both healthcare providers and consumers and a trend toward short-term, solution-focused treatment plans which are deemed more expedient in terms of cost, time and demands on personnel. It is unlikely that these trends in managed care can respond to the needs of patients suffering from eating disorders. Treatment is often long-term, complicated and demanding. The patient-centered approach provides a positive framework for understanding and guiding the management of eating disorders, one that offers renewed hope for both sufferers and their families.

# Reference

Stewart M, Brown JB, Weston WW *et al.* (1995) *Patient-Centered Medicine: transforming the clinical method.* Sage Publications, Thousand Oaks, CA.

# Index